THE
ENERGY BOOSTER
WORKOUT

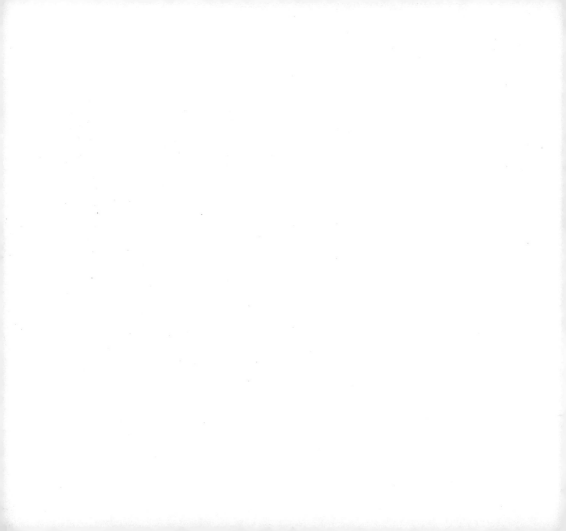

THE ENERGY BOOSTER WORKOUT

SIMON BROWN

Illustrated by
IAN DICKS

Marlowe & Company
New York

PLEASE NOTE

The author, packager and publisher cannot accept any responsibility for misadventure
resulting from the practice of any of the exercises set out in this book. Please refer to a
medical professional if you are in any doubt about any aspect of your condition.

Published in the United States by Marlowe and Company
An Imprint of Avalon Publishing Group Incorporated
161 William Street, Sixteenth Floor, New York, NY 10038
Distributed by Publishers Group West

ISBN 1-56924-442-1
Library of Congress Control Number: 2003106895

1   3   5   7   9   10   8   6   4   2

AN EDDISON·SADD EDITION
Edited, Designed and Produced by
Eddison Sadd Editions Limited
St Chad's House, 148 King's Cross Road
London WC1X 9DH

Phototypeset in The Mix, HF Doodle and Gill using QuarkXPress on Apple Macintosh
Origination by Pixel Tech, Singapore
Printed by Kyodo Printing Co., Singapore

CONTENTS

FOREWORD

When Dan Fletcher and I first thought of this book back in 1990 we wanted to create something unique that would make feeling good easy and fun. I was the director of the Community Health Foundation in London and regularly teaching 'Do In' and shiatsu, while Dan had a successful career producing cartoon manuals teaching people how to do anything from cleaning a train to operating a crane.

The book sold in its thousands and soon became something of a cult phenomenon. Everyone loved the fact that it did not feature super-slim models and that it was unpretentious, funny and easy to follow. But most importantly people kept coming back to buy more copies for their friends because they found that the exercises worked and made them feel better.

Now, I am excited that this new version is being published, with brand new illustrations by Ian Dicks. I have re-written much of the text to bring it up to date and to include all the experience I have gained since the original version was produced. I very much hope you enjoy it.

INTRODUCTION

The exercises in this book combine simple stretches and loosening-up exercises with the massage of special acupressure points. These self-massage exercises are derived from ancient Japanese exercises, known collectively as 'Do In'. I have integrated the two types of exercises to provide an all-round workout that will make you feel energized and relaxed at the same time. You should feel a buzz of energy in your body, which will also feel lighter, freer, more flexible and stretched out. I hope you will also be aware of a sensation of calm and clear-headedness.

GET FLEXIBLE

In traditional Oriental medicine one of the prime indicators of good health is flexibility. The body has a natural elasticity self-evident in youth. Unfortunately, as the body ages it tends to become both less flexible and more loose as it loses its elasticity. Your bones, internal organs, skin, muscles, tendons and ligaments all suffer in this way.

This particular combination of exercises, and the order in which they are included in the book, is designed to help you retain, or regain, your natural elasticity and delay the ageing process.

This book enables you to work through a wide range of stretches and

Do In exercises easily. The exercises cover a wide range of techniques, including stretching, pounding, massaging, applying pressure, rocking, breathing and meditation. Together they make up a routine that has plenty of variety and cannot fail to boost your energy.

ROUTINES FOR EVERYONE

Once you are familiar with the exercises you may like to use the at-a-glance programmes that begin on page 146. In this section, a visual reminder of all the exercises is displayed for the full programme, which takes around 45 minutes, together with a 25-minute and a 10-minute routine. So, even if you are very pressed for time, you have no excuse not to do some kind of exercise routine every day. Towards the end of the book there is a small selection of stretches and shiatsu exercises for two people who want to work out together. I have also written some more detailed information about Oriental approaches to exercise and diet.

BEFORE YOU START

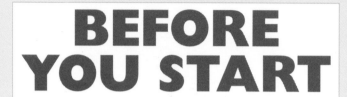

This section shows you how to really get to know yourself in a way that allows you to become much more intuitive about what is good for you. Here you will find a way of talking and listening to your body that means you can take action before you start to suffer from bodily aches and pains.

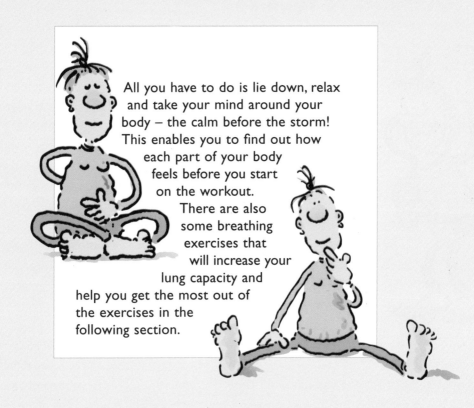

All you have to do is lie down, relax and take your mind around your body – the calm before the storm! This enables you to find out how each part of your body feels before you start on the workout. There are also some breathing exercises that will increase your lung capacity and help you get the most out of the exercises in the following section.

Throughout the evolution of humankind survival has always depended on strong instincts about what and when to eat and drink, when to work and when to relax. Sadly, in modern life, many of these healthy instincts have become dulled.

How often do you drink when you are not thirsty, eat when you are not hungry, sit around when you need to move, or overwork when you should take time out and relax? It's time to pay more attention to your body.

To be naturally healthy you need to listen closely and accurately to your body's needs and act upon that information. For example, you should drink when you feel thirsty, and you should eat when you feel hungry – and not at any other times. Similarly, you you should take time out to relax or go to sleep when your body tells you that it is tired. If you pay attention, your body can even tell you when to exercise and stretch your muscles.

BECOMING ACQUAINTED

By listening to your body you can become more in touch with your needs, and know more exactly how to look after yourself.

Over the following eight pages you will find some simple relaxation and listening exercises designed to help you get in touch with your body and attune to its needs. By doing these exercises regularly you will get to know your body really well and develop the intuition to know exactly what you need.

Developing this intuition helps you know what works for you and what doesn't. Use it to test the effectiveness of the exercises in this book!

RELAX AND FOCUS

We are all good at recognizing pain or discomfort but not so used to sensing the state of the body when there is no real crisis. The following exercise enables you to improve this ability. It involves taking your mind around your whole body, focusing intently on each part in turn. By so doing you subconsciously send a shaft of mental energy to each area, helping you to heal and improve the well-being of your entire body.

By doing this exercise regularly, you can more accurately monitor the subtle daily changes that occur in your body. You can then use this information to prevent anything more serious going wrong.

Although the exercise is shown being done lying down, in fact you can do it equally well sitting up. This means you can do it anywhere. A bus, train or café will all work fine. Take any opportunity you can to get to know your body.

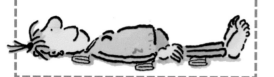

WARNING!

If you feel any discomfort, use a towel or cushion to make yourself comfortable. If it helps, put a support under your neck, lower back or your knees.

GET COMFORTABLE

Before you start, make sure you won't be disturbed for half an hour. Lie on your back on a firm flat surface.

CONCENTRATE

During the exercise, try to feel each part of your body as you concentrate on it. If you find it hard to keep up concentration, focus your mind on each part of your body by addressing it with the question I suggest on the following pages.

Imagine on each out-breath that you are breathing energy into the part of the body that you are concentrating on and take your mind there. Be attentive to every detail, however small.

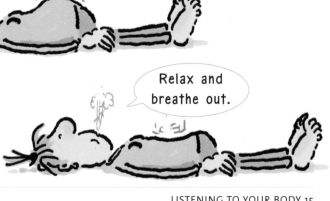

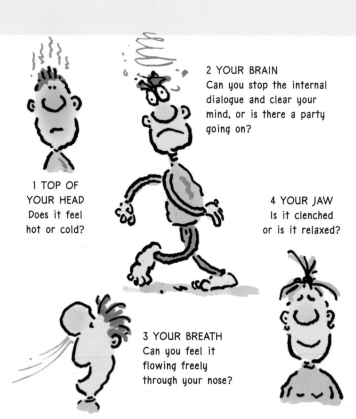

WHAT TO DO

Focus your mind on each part of your body in turn, from head to toe – ideally while lying down. Use the questions provided to help you. I often do this before and after an exercise to find out how that exercise has benefited my body. It is also interesting to do it before and after work, or before a meal and again an hour after to find out whether what you ate was healthy for you.

1 TOP OF YOUR HEAD
Does it feel hot or cold?

2 YOUR BRAIN
Can you stop the internal dialogue and clear your mind, or is there a party going on?

4 YOUR JAW
Is it clenched or is it relaxed?

3 YOUR BREATH
Can you feel it flowing freely through your nose?

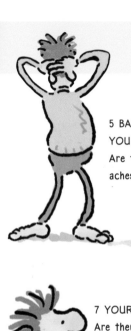

5 BACK OF YOUR HEAD
Are there any aches or pains?

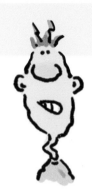

6 YOUR NECK
Is it stiff or relaxed?

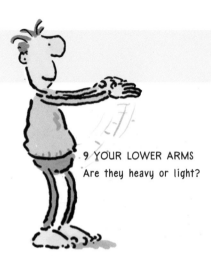

9 YOUR LOWER ARMS
Are they heavy or light?

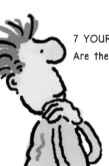

7 YOUR SHOULDERS
Are they relaxed or painful?

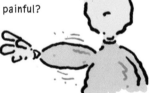

8 YOUR UPPER ARMS
Are they tired or energetic?

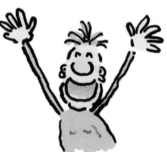

10 YOUR HANDS
Are they hot, cold, dry or damp?

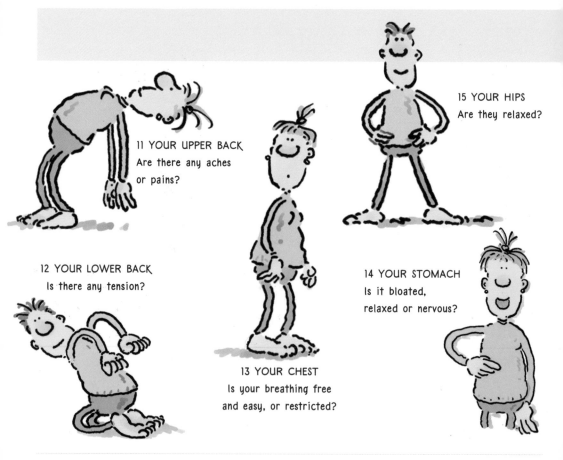

11 YOUR UPPER BACK
Are there any aches
or pains?

12 YOUR LOWER BACK
Is there any tension?

13 YOUR CHEST
Is your breathing free
and easy, or restricted?

14 YOUR STOMACH
Is it bloated,
relaxed or nervous?

15 YOUR HIPS
Are they relaxed?

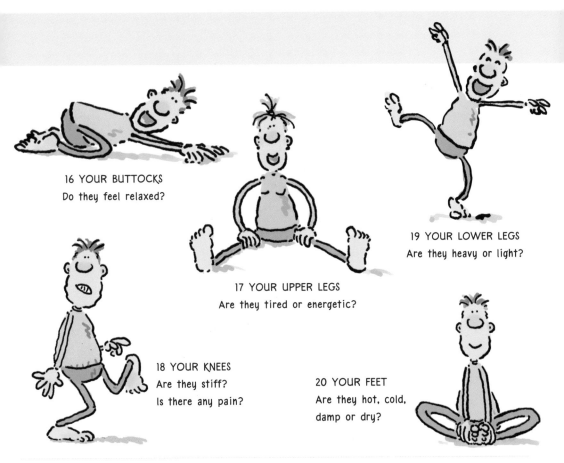

16 YOUR BUTTOCKS
Do they feel relaxed?

17 YOUR UPPER LEGS
Are they tired or energetic?

18 YOUR KNEES
Are they stiff?
Is there any pain?

19 YOUR LOWER LEGS
Are they heavy or light?

20 YOUR FEET
Are they hot, cold,
damp or dry?

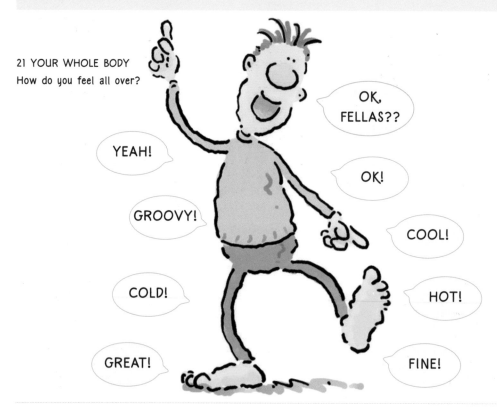

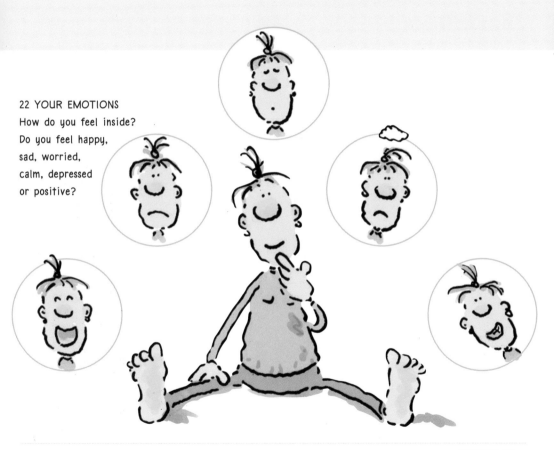

22 YOUR EMOTIONS
How do you feel inside?
Do you feel happy,
sad, worried,
calm, depressed
or positive?

BREATHING

We are more dependent on breathing than on any other bodily function. If we do not breathe for seven minutes we will die. Yet breathing is something we usually pay very little attention to.

WORKING WITH THE BREATH

Try breathing out as you lift something heavy, or as you push open a heavy, spring-loaded door. You will find that the action seems easier if you do it on the out-breath. In shiatsu massage, I often notice that as my patient breathes out, his or her body relaxes more and it is possible to stretch further. Try breathing out as you stretch and see for yourself. After a while you may find working with the breath becomes second nature.

Students of the martial arts are advised to 'breathe from the abdomen', which means trying to breathe so that your abdomen expands with your in-breath and contracts with your out-breath. This helps to massage the internal organs and increases your breathing capacity. In addition, martial arts practitioners find that such exercises have the effect of lowering the centre of gravity and increasing inner strength.

BREATHING EXERCISE

To help keep your respiratory system fit see how much air you can breathe into your lungs and then try to fully empty them. As you first breathe in, push the air down, as though into your abdomen. Then fill the chest and finally raise your arms up and back to completely fill yourself with air. As you breathe out, tighten the muscles in the abdomen to squeeze out as much air as you can.

BREATHING FROM THE ABDOMEN

1. Place one hand over your navel and the other hand behind your back. Feel your abdomen expand as you breathe in.
2. As you breathe out, contract the abdomen and feel the hands come together.

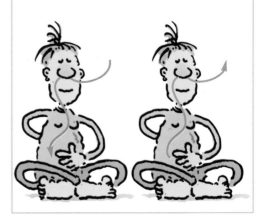

GETTING READY

This section of the book shows you how to loosen and warm up your body in preparation for the main workout. This ensures that you do not strain any part of your body later and that you get the most out of the workout because you feel relaxed. After the warm-up exercises I demonstrate how to generate healing energy in your hands. You will need this energy to massage and apply pressure to each part of your body when you get to the main section of the book.

LOOSEN-UP SHAKES

WHAT TO DO

Imagine you are going to shake the blood all around your body and get your circulation buzzing.

Plant your feet securely on the floor so you have good balance. Start with one arm and shake it vigorously. Try to make the shake start from your shoulder and move all the way to the tips of your fingers. Do the same for your other arm. Now move on to your legs. Lift one leg off the ground and shake it, starting from your hip and letting the shake become wilder as it reaches the tips of your toes. Do the same with the other leg. Finally, bounce up and down, shaking arms and legs at the same time.

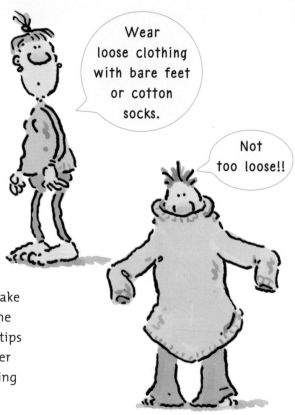

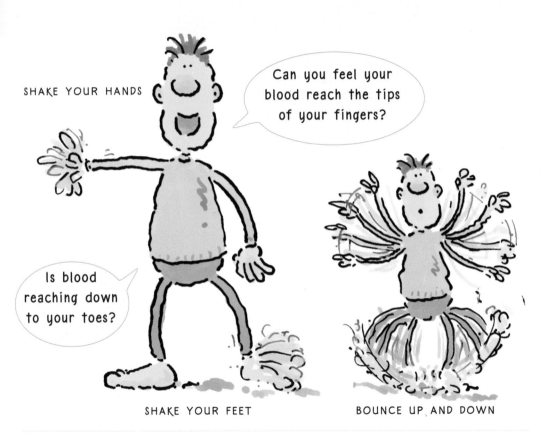

SIDE-TO-SIDE FLOPS

Repeat 10 times

Standing with legs shoulder-width apart and knees slightly bent ...

... swing round from the hips, letting your arms flop around the body to the left ...

... looking behind you as far as you can.

WHAT TO DO

In this exercise you twist all the knots out of your back and free up your shoulders. Bounce on your knees and adjust your feet until you feel you are firmly connected with the ground. Bend your knees and use your hips to start a twisting motion from side to side. Make your arms as floppy as possible so they spin out on each turn, then slap against your body as you change direction.

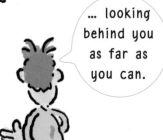

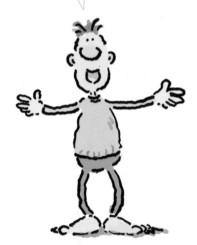

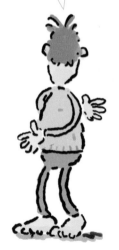

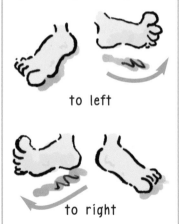

TIP FOR STIFF HIPS

If your hip joints are painful when you turn, pivot your left foot as you turn left and your right foot as you turn right.

to left

to right

REACH FOR THE STARS

Stand up straight, legs together, arms by your sides.

Breathing in, step forward with the left leg and stretch towards the sky.

WHAT TO DO

This is an excellent stretch for opening up your lungs and stretching out the muscles, tendons and ligaments of your upper body. It is ideal if you have been sitting at a computer or in a car for too long. As you stretch up, your chest opens, creating more space for your lungs to expand into, improving their elasticity.

This stretch helps you free up your upper body to make it easier to generate a healing energy in your hands later. You should feel a weight lifted from your shoulders after you have worked through this sequence.

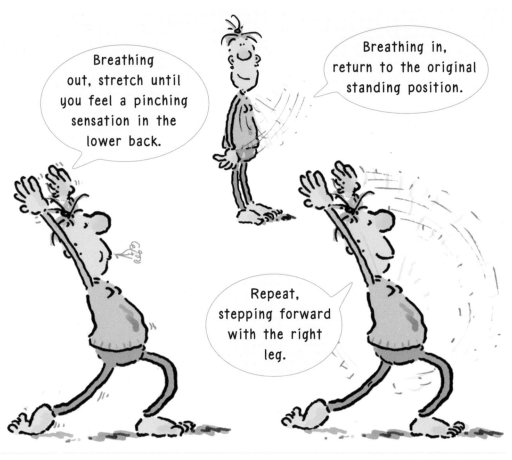

WINDMILL ARMS

WHAT TO DO

This exercise will help your shoulders feel looser and reduce any loss of mobility as you get older. The idea is to rotate your arms and move your shoulders without using your shoulder muscles. Use your knees to move your spine and start a swinging action in both your arms. Once you get a rhythm going, see how far you can swing your arms.

The shoulders are very loose joints, so you should find you can move them easily. If you feel up to it, try fully spinning one arm at a time using the same swinging movement.

Swing your arms backwards and forwards ...

... bending your knees as your arms go down.

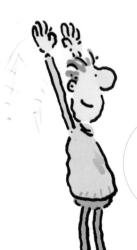

Straighten your legs as your arms go up.

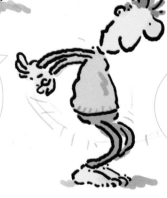

Then go into full arm rotation, using the body to swing one arm. Repeat with the other arm.

... without using arm or shoulder muscles.

Repeat until you have a good swinging motion ...

SHOULDER–BODY STRETCH

WHAT TO DO

Here you get another chance to open up your lungs. This time you stretch forward, compressing your lungs slightly and making it easier to get all the air out of your system. You also give all the soft tissues in your shoulders a stretch and work on your abdomen. You will probably be amazed at how far you can bend your body in each direction.

This exercise frees up the healing energy associated with your lungs and intestines. It helps you get energy from your abdomen into your upper body where you will need it to develop and focus the healing powers in your hands.

Place hands behind back and link thumbs.

Push both arms up to the sky ...

BREATHE OUT

... hold for 6 seconds ...

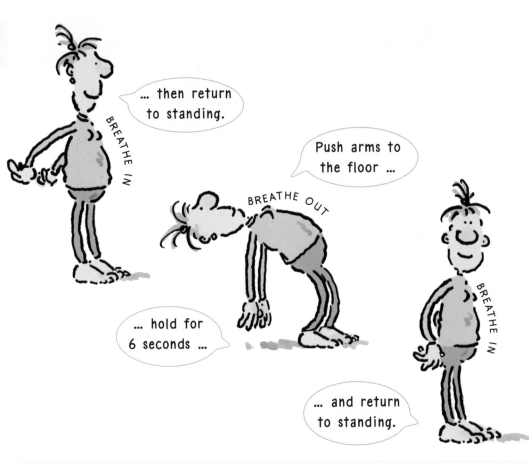

CHANGING YOUR CHI ENERGY

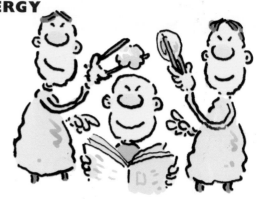

Central to traditional Oriental medicine is the belief that a subtle 'life-energy', called chi or ki, flows through every organism along invisible pathways known as meridians. Each meridian line takes energy to a particular organ or part of the body.

In my experience this flow of energy can be altered by pressing certain acupressure points, which are located in specific places along each meridian line. Meridian charts describe 360 such points on the human body. In acupuncture, each point has a particular purpose and is used to treat specific health problems. Massaging the points can also provide pain relief, as this action releases endorphins. In China, this technique is sometimes used during surgery instead of anaesthetics.

Acupressure points are often used for diagnosis. If you feel an unpleasant sickening pain when pressure is applied to a particular point on a meridian line, then you probably need to improve the condition of the related organ. Sometimes a point that initially feels sore will improve simply by pressing it.

HOW TO CULTIVATE CHI ENERGY

This exercise increases your chi energy and encourages a good amount of it to move into your hands. There it will give your hands a healing power when you use them to press acupressure points in specific exercises in the workout. Repeat six times.

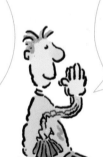

With an empty mind, imagine a fire roaring in your abdomen. As you breathe in, visualize the flames being fanned.

As you breathe out — contracting your abdomen — imagine the flames travelling up and into your hands.

GETTING YOUR HANDS READY

WHAT TO DO

This is where you start to concentrate your healing energy, or chi, in your hands. It is an incredible sensation when you get it right.

You can do this preparatory exercise in a kneeling, sitting or standing position – whichever works best for you. The main thing is to relax and let it all happen naturally. If you force it and get tense you will end up restricting your flow of chi, making it harder to get the energy flowing into your hands.

Kneel, stand or sit – whichever is most comfortable.

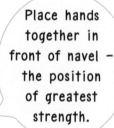

Place hands together in front of navel – the position of greatest strength.

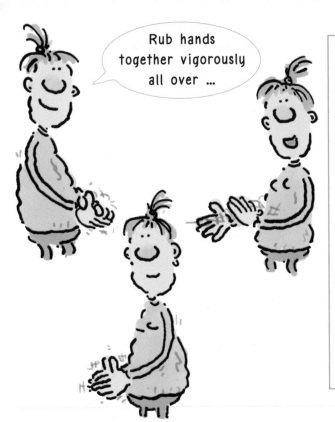

INCREASE YOUR HAND POWER

Your hands are strongest when placed just in front of your navel. Next time you need to unscrew the tight lid of a jar, hold the jar in in front of your navel to feel how much easier it is to open in this position. For greater power in your hands, use this position as the starting point for as many movements as possible.

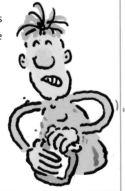

Move your hands together and apart slowly, while continuing to breathe and focus on the imagery of chi filling your abdomen and flowing up to your hands. Try closing your eyes for greater sensitivity.

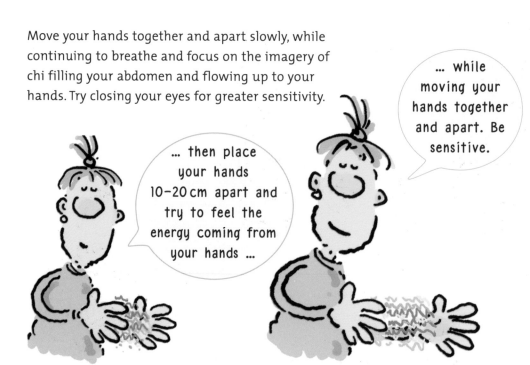

... then place your hands 10–20 cm apart and try to feel the energy coming from your hands ...

... while moving your hands together and apart. Be sensitive.

FINGER WORKOUT

WHAT TO DO

This exercise draws out and extends your chi energy field around your fingers. It involves massaging, rotating and pulling each finger of each hand in turn to draw up chi from deep inside your body, stimulating a freeing-up of energy all along the finger meridians. Hold your hands in front of your navel and begin by taking the forefinger of one hand between the thumb and forefinger of the other. When you have completed the exercise your fingers should be radiating long flames of chi.

At the base of a finger, hold each side between thumb and forefinger.

Twist and pull, rubbing along the finger to the tip.

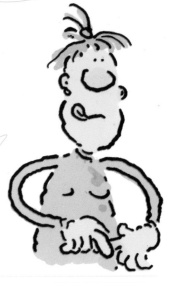

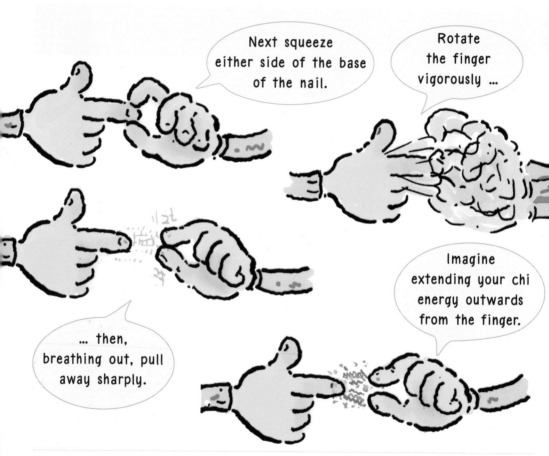

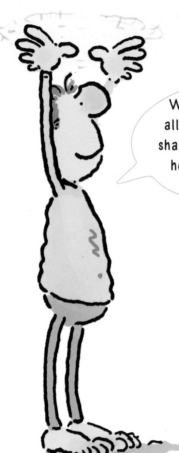

When you have exercised all the fingers and thumbs, shake your hands above your head — imagine polishing the sky!

TIP OF THE ICEBERG

In Chinese medicine the tips of the most peripheral part of the body – the fingers and toes – are exercised to stimulate or relax deep inside the torso.

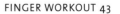

WORKOUT FOR ONE

Now you have the chi energy radiating from your hands you are ready to apply it to yourself. This is where you start the self-healing process of getting your chi to move harmoniously around your body.

Here you will discover how to calm your mind while making your body more energetic. The loosening-up and pressure-point exercises are carefully organized to give your whole body a thorough but safe workout in one routine that takes around 45 minutes. If you don't have time to complete the whole workout, turn to the Programmes section (page 146) for alternative shorter routines. Information about the acupressure points and meridians you are working on is included with each Do In exercise, to help you understand what you are doing.

This section is where it all happens and I hope you feel the difference!

These illustrations show the location of the acupressure points on the meridians that run through the hand and arm, and the organs related to each. When trying to locate a particular acupressure point, move the thumb around the area until you feel the greatest effect. The point may feel sore or you may feel a sharp pain or tingling sensation when you press it deeply. When you have found the point, lightly massage with your thumb as you breathe in and then press on it for about five seconds as you breathe out. Press any one point three times unless it is particularly sensitive, in which case spend longer on it.

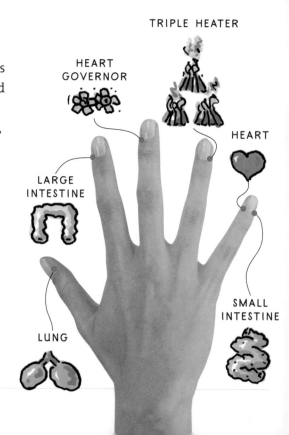

TRIPLE HEATER

HEART GOVERNOR

HEART

LARGE INTESTINE

SMALL INTESTINE

LUNG

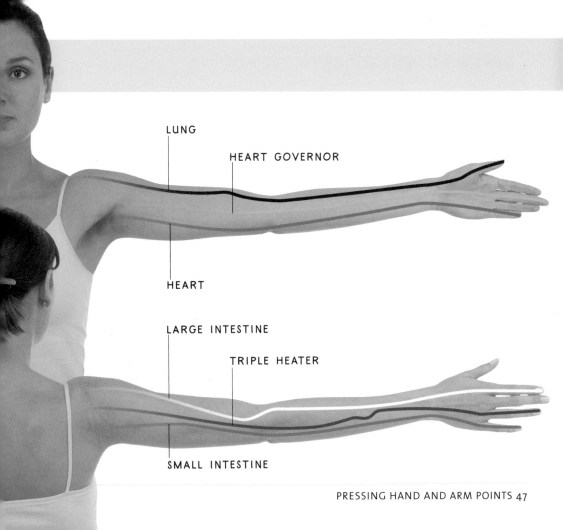

LUNG

HEART GOVERNOR

HEART

LARGE INTESTINE

TRIPLE HEATER

SMALL INTESTINE

WHAT TO DO

You can massage hand and arm acupressure points sitting down, kneeling or standing – whatever is most comfortable for you. The points can be found next to ridges in your bones, in indentations in your soft tissues or at a crease in a joint. You will know when you have found one as it will be sensitive to the touch. First locate the general area, then press on it with your thumb, making a circling motion as you look for the exact spot. Always do the equivalent points on both sides of the body – for example, on the left and right hands.

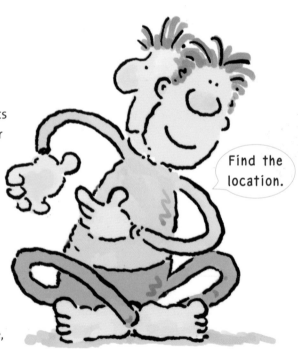

Find the location.

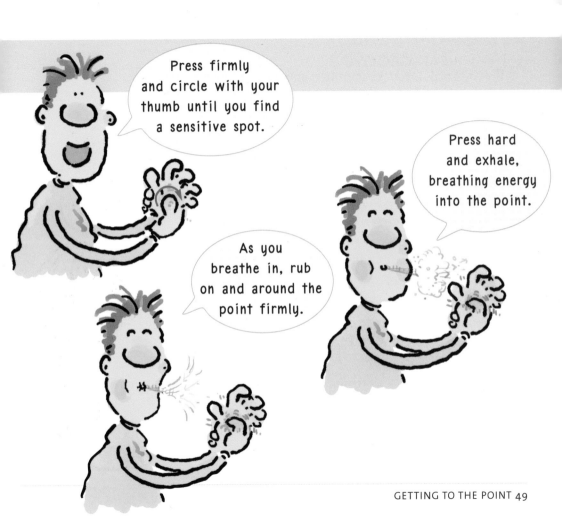

WHAT TO DO

This is a good point to press for relieving abdominal pains. To locate the point find the bone that runs down the side of your hand from your little finger. Slide your thumb up and down this bone. About half-way down you will find a small indentation in the bone. Press into the indentation firmly and edge up and down. If you press hard enough you will find a point that will trigger a fairly sharp pain. This is the spot! Remember the feeling you get when you have hit the spot to make it easier to find in the future.

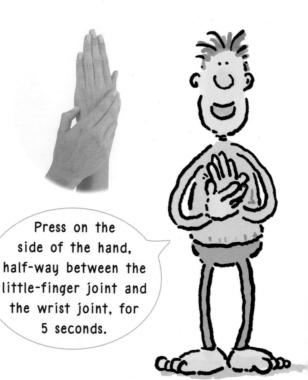

Press on the side of the hand, half-way between the little-finger joint and the wrist joint, for 5 seconds.

DIGESTIVE
DISORDERS AND
ABDOMINAL
PAIN

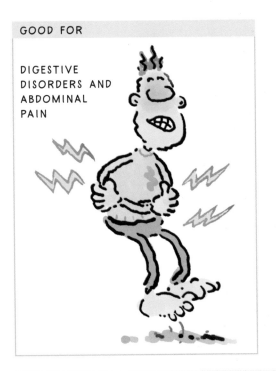

SMALL INTESTINE
MERIDIAN (yang)

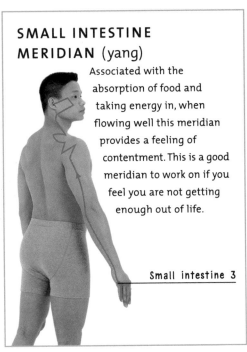

Associated with the
absorption of food and
taking energy in, when
flowing well this meridian
provides a feeling of
contentment. This is a good
meridian to work on if you
feel you are not getting
enough out of life.

Small intestine 3

WHAT TO DO

This is a great point for stimulating endorphins, the body's natural pain killer. To find it, press into the fleshy part between your thumb and finger. Rub the bone that leads from your first finger to the joint with your thumb. About half-way along you will find a small notch in the bone. Put your fingers on the other side of the flesh so that you can press firmly with your thumb. You will know when you have found it as it will be painful! Rub to release endorphins or press to nourish your intestines.

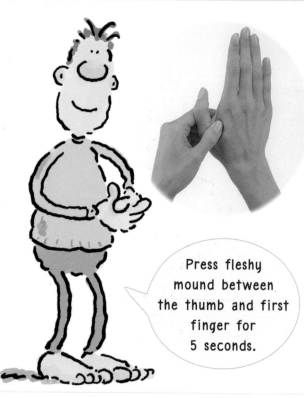

Press fleshy mound between the thumb and first finger for 5 seconds.

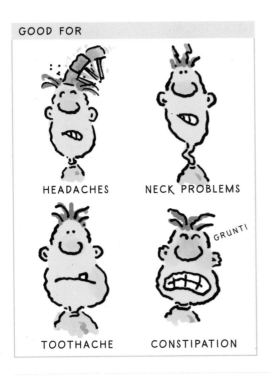

GOOD FOR

HEADACHES

NECK PROBLEMS

TOOTHACHE

CONSTIPATION

GRUNT!

LARGE INTESTINE MERIDIAN (yang)

Responsible for the elimination of solid waste and re-absorption of liquids, the chi energy in this meridian is good for keeping things moving. When this energy does not flow well, the person concerned often becomes withdrawn.

Large intestine 11

Large intestine 4

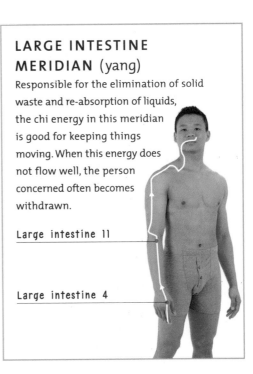

LAKE OF ENERGY ON THE CORNER
Large intestine meridian point 11

Repeat 3 times
on each elbow

WHAT TO DO

Energy can often get stuck in joints, and pressing this point will help you get energy moving throughout your arm. Bend your elbow to a right angle so that it forms a crease. Press firmly into the end of the crease. Rotate your thumb slowly until you find a sensitive point. Press carefully for 5 seconds on each out-breath.

Press at the end of the crease in the elbow when arm bent at right angles for 5 seconds.

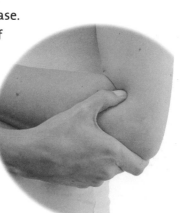

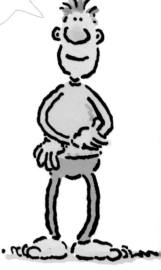

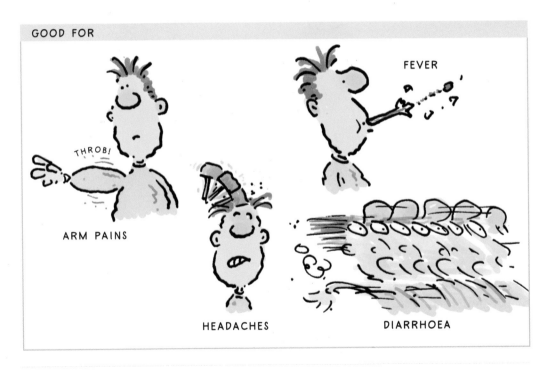

WHAT TO DO

This is the point to press if you feel any kind of nausea. To find it, slide your thumb about 4 cm (1½ in) down from the centre of the inside of your wrist. Press into the groove between the two tendons and look for a sharp pain by sliding your thumb up and down slightly. Press in as deeply as possible while breathing out. If you are feeling really sick you will have to work quite hard into the point on both wrists to feel any benefit.

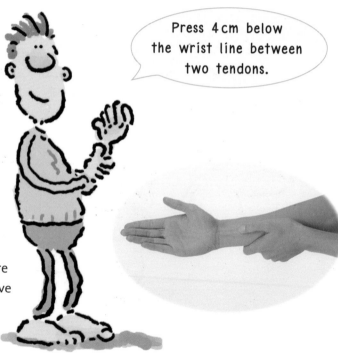

Press 4 cm below the wrist line between two tendons.

GOOD FOR

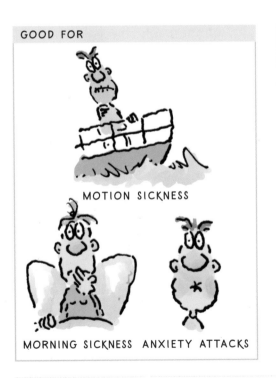

MOTION SICKNESS

MORNING SICKNESS   ANXIETY ATTACKS

HEART GOVERNOR MERIDIAN (yin)

Although this does not relate directly to the heart, the energy within this meridian is instrumental in blood circulation. Enhancing this flow of energy creates a calming feeling and relieves stress. It will also help you get rid of stagnation in your body or your life.

Heart governor 6

Heart governor 8

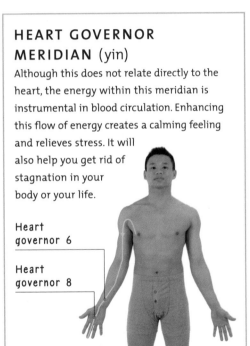

PALACE OF EXHAUSTION
Heart governor meridian point 8

Repeat 3 times on each hand

WHAT TO DO

Pressing on this point will help build up your overall energy levels. To find the point, clench your hand into a fist and observe where your longest finger contacts the palm of your hand. Open your hand and press into this point with your thumb. As you press, let your hand relax and close a little so that it is easier to let your thumb sink into the flesh. Circle around until you find a dull ache. When you have found this acupressure point, breathe chi energy into it strongly.

Press in the middle of the palm (the point just below the middle finger when your fingers are clenched) for 5 seconds.

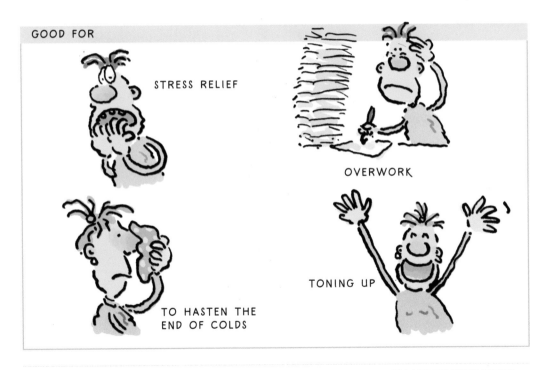

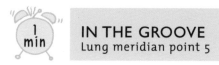
WHAT TO DO

This is a good point to press to alleviate all kinds of respiratory problems. Bend your elbow to 90 degrees so that you have a deep crease on the inside of your elbow. Place your thumb on the crease on the inside of your forearm muscle. Straighten your arm and slide your thumb one thumb-width towards your hand. Holding the outside of your muscle with your fingers, slide the flat of your thumb towards and away from your elbow along the muscle until you find the exact spot.

> Open arm out straight. At the point just below the elbow crease, squeeze the forearm muscle for 5 seconds.

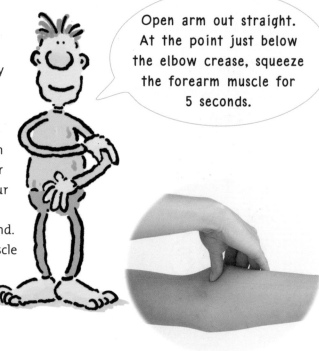

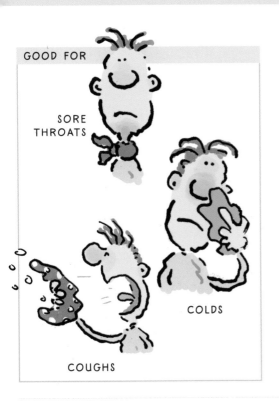

GOOD FOR

SORE THROATS

COLDS

COUGHS

LUNG MERIDIAN (yin)

This meridian is responsible for the absorption of oxygen and the elimination of carbon monoxide. It is also influential in the body's ability to take in chi energy. Good energy flow along this meridian fosters positive thinking and physical endurance. When this energy is weak it becomes easier to feel depressed.

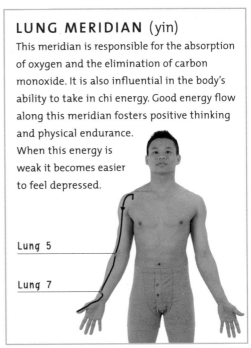

Lung 5

Lung 7

BROKEN SEQUENCE
Lung meridian point 7

Repeat 3 times on each arm

WHAT TO DO

If you're feeling bunged up and run down, this is a good point to press to clear your head and perk you up. Place your fingers on the inside of your wrist so that the little finger fits neatly into the groove of your wrist. Look at the place where your index finger falls on the inside of your forearm. Press onto the bone that leads to your thumb with your thumb and slide it up and down until you find a sensitive indentation.

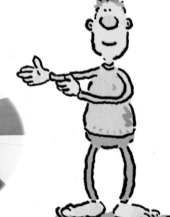

Press 4 fingers along from the wrist on the inside top of the arm for 5 seconds.

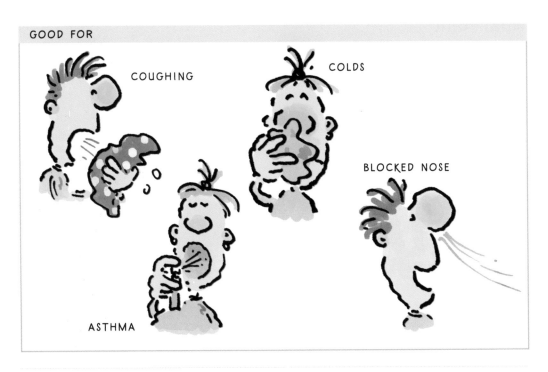

WHAT TO DO

Pressing this point is particularly good for restoring a sense of calm in times of distress or panic.

Look at the inside of your wrist and bend it slightly so that you can see a crease. Place your thumb on the crease so that it is in line with your little finger. Feel around to find a bony protrusion. Press the tip of your thumb just inside this bone to find the point. As you rub up and down you should feel a sharp sensation. The point can be a little difficult to find, so you may need to press quite hard and at different angles, exploring the area a little, to hit the right spot.

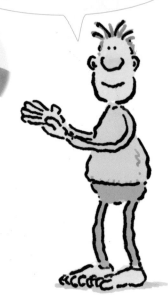

Press on the wrist line on the inside of the bony knob for 5 seconds.

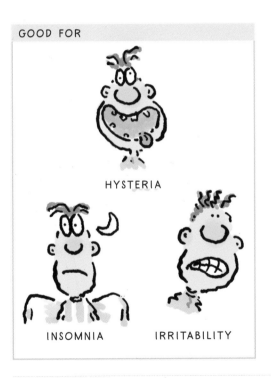

HYSTERIA

INSOMNIA

IRRITABILITY

HEART MERIDIAN (yin)

The energy along this meridian gives us our spirit of adventure and provides us with a sense of rhythm. When out of balance, you are likely to feel slightly hysterical or panicky. When the energy is flowing well along this meridian you feel you have plenty of fighting spirit and that your sense of timing is spot on.

Heart 7

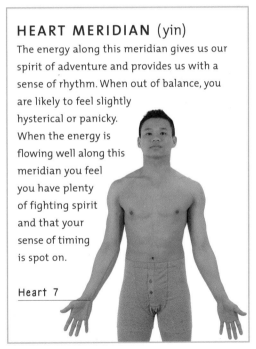

CREATING WARMTH
Triple heater meridian

WHAT TO DO

To create warmth throughout your body, you need to stimulate the triple heater meridian. The best way to do this is to rub the outside of each arm vigorously in turn. Press quite hard, so you can feel the palms of your hands getting hot. Include the backs of your hands and the tops of your shoulders when you are rubbing. You should begin to feel a warmth move through your whole body after a minute or so. You might even feel a mild buzz in your body as the chi in this meridian becomes more active.

> Rub the top of the arm up and down 10 times.

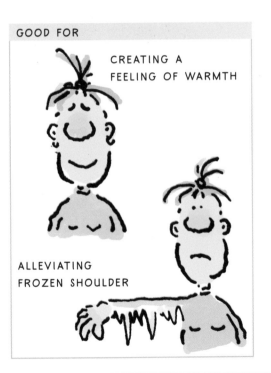

CREATING A
FEELING OF WARMTH

ALLEVIATING
FROZEN SHOULDER

TRIPLE HEATER MERIDIAN (yang)

This meridian runs through the three areas at the front of the torso where energy is created out of food, water and air, creating warmth and energy. When this energy is working well you will find that you combine your food, water and air efficiently to produce maximum energy.

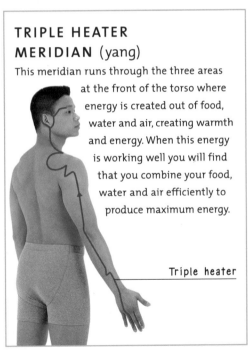

Triple heater

PRESSING AND RUBBING HEAD AND FACE POINTS

These illustrations show the location of the meridians that run through the head, and the organs related to each. Some meridian lines travel the full length of your body. These include the stomach, bladder and gall bladder meridians, which run all the way up from the toes. You can therefore work anywhere along these meridian lines to change – for example – the chi in your head. This is why you can calm a headache by working on your feet.

In addition, the large intestine, small intestine and triple heater meridians run from your fingers into your head, so large intestine 4 in your hand is also useful in reducing pains in your head.

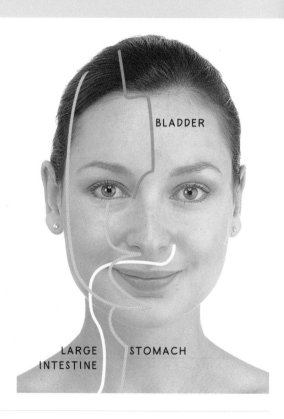

BLADDER

LARGE INTESTINE

STOMACH

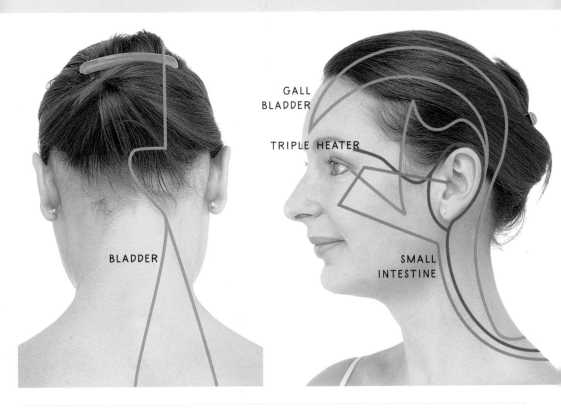

GALL
BLADDER

TRIPLE HEATER

SMALL
INTESTINE

BLADDER

WHAT TO DO

Before trying to locate a particular pressure point on your head or face, you need to really get to know your skull. Take some time to seek out those slightly painful indentations and ridges.

Many of these points will respond well to rubbing or to a circular motion. Also, try pressing on them for a while as you concentrate on breathing chi into the whole meridian.

You might find it easier to do the face exercises in front of a mirror so you can see what you are doing and find the points more easily.

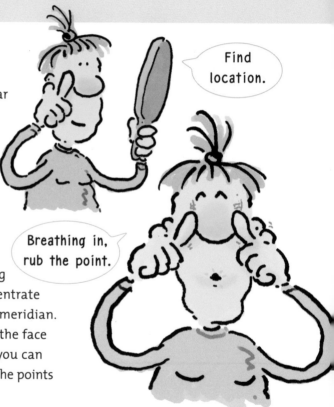

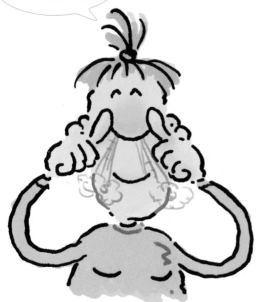

Press point, breathing out for 5 seconds.

IT'S IN YOUR FACE

The way your chi moves through your face will alter your facial expressions and, with age, even change your appearance. When I give a shiatsu massage I see the person's face change as I work on their hands and feet. Essentially, if you have a light, responsive chi it will show in your face, and people will warm to you easily.

WELCOME FRAGRANCE
Large intestine meridian point 20

WHAT TO DO

This is an excellent point for helping your breathing. Place your index fingers either side of the base of your nostrils and press in, circling to get the tips of your fingers into a small hollow in the bones. This may be quite painful, so you will need to work into it slowly to activate the point and get fresh chi into the meridian.

For a blocked nose, press the point firmly on either side and then, as you breathe out, slide your fingers out across your cheeks, all the way to your ears, applying as much pressure as possible.

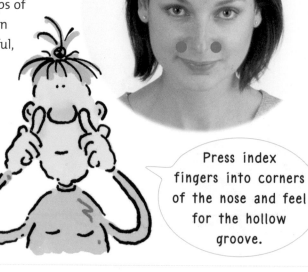

Press index fingers into corners of the nose and feel for the hollow groove.

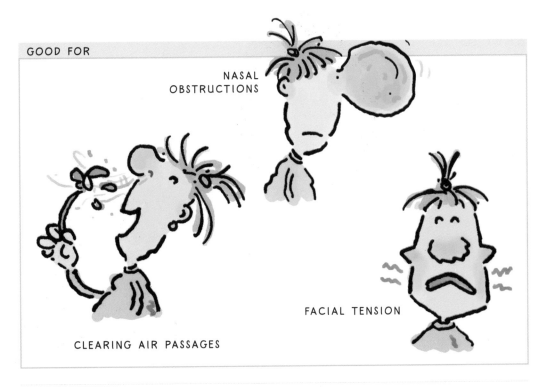

GOOD FOR

NASAL OBSTRUCTIONS

CLEARING AIR PASSAGES

FACIAL TENSION

WHAT TO DO

This point is helpful in draining your sinuses, or any sinus-related problems. Follow it up by rubbing vigorously around your eyes and lightly pounding your forehead.

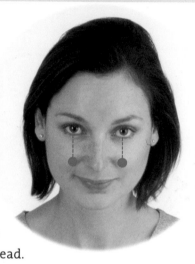

Looking in the mirror, slide your thumbs down from your eyes until you locate a hollow at the bottom of your cheekbones. Your thumbs should be in line with your nostrils. Circle your thumbs in the hollow until you find the most sensitive area. Then breathe chi into the point.

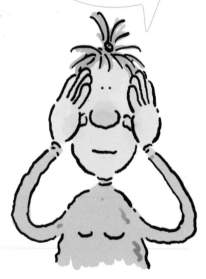

Press with your thumbs into the hollow below the cheekbones. This is directly below the pupils when looking ahead.

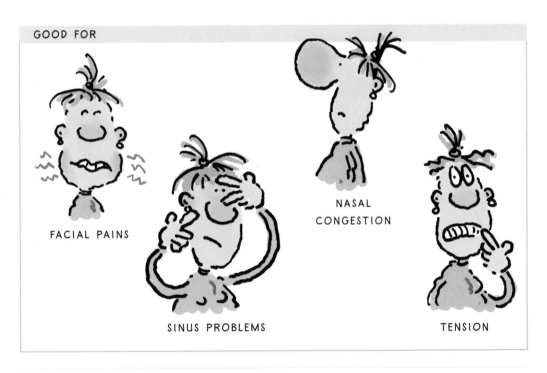

GOOD FOR

FACIAL PAINS

SINUS PROBLEMS

NASAL CONGESTION

TENSION

WHAT TO DO

Good for alleviating headaches, this acupressure point is not easy to work on. However, by letting your head drop forwards slightly and using your fingers to grip the top of your skull, you can apply pressure to it successfully.

Look for a ridge at the base of the back of your skull. Using your thumbs, slide out from the centre until you cross the main tendons running under the ridge. Just outside these tendons you will find two hollows in the ridge.

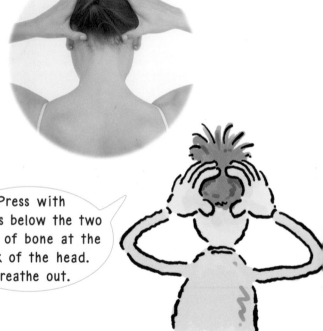

Press with thumbs below the two lumps of bone at the back of the head. Breathe out.

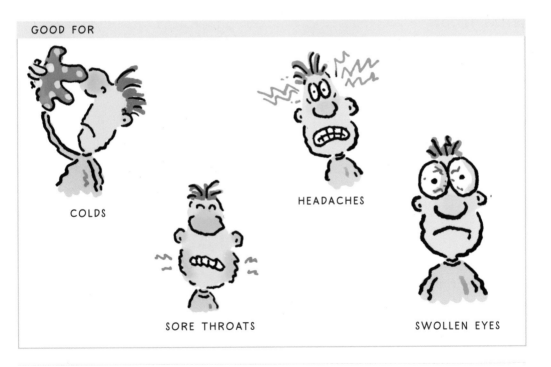

GOOD FOR

COLDS

SORE THROATS

HEADACHES

SWOLLEN EYES

HEAD AND FACE MASSAGE 1

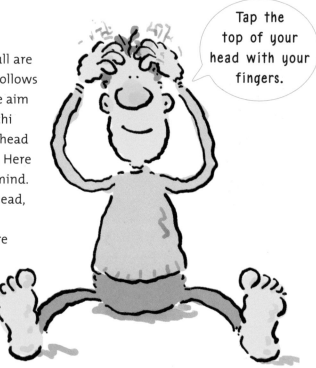

Tap the top of your head with your fingers.

WHAT TO DO

The bones that make up your skull are full of ridges, indentations and hollows where chi can easily get stuck. The aim of this exercise is to get all that chi flowing freely again so that your head feels fresh, clear and invigorated. Here is your chance to clear out your mind.

As you massage around your head, look out for all those interesting contours in your bones and be sure to work into them carefully. Don't worry if you get sidetracked from the sequence for a while if you find a place that needs attention.

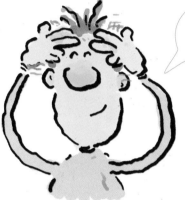

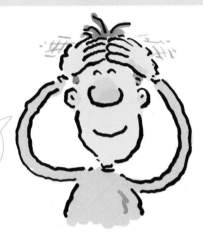

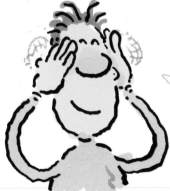

HEAD AND FACE MASSAGE 2

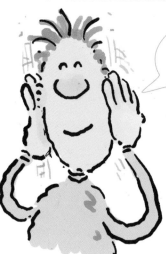

Rub your cheeks up and down vigorously. This is good for waking up and increasing your energy.

Rub the sides of your nose up and down vigorously.

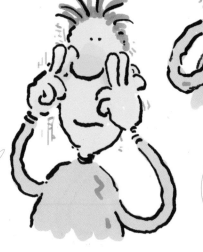

Squeeze along jaw bone. This is good for relaxation and stimulating saliva glands.

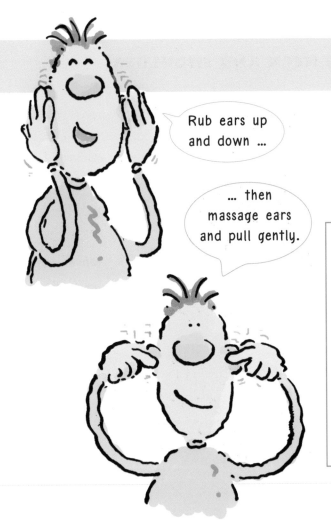

ORIENTAL WISDOM

The Chinese regard large ears with good lobes as a sign of a strong constitution. Take a close look at those who have abused their bodies but survived. Do they have large ears and fulsome lobes?

MASSAGING NECK AND SHOULDERS

WHAT TO DO

This massage dissolves stress, helps align muscle fibre and increases the flow of blood. It also removes waste products, such as lactic acid. The idea is to squeeze all the toxins and waste out of these muscles.

Try squeezing the muscles as firmly as possible while moving your head around, so that you can feel the muscles moving under your hand. If you can grip them strongly enough to stop the muscles moving you can give yourself a good massage by simply moving your head around.

> Grasp the back of the neck with the palm of the hand, squeeze firmly and massage.

> Move the head around into different positions. Repeat with the other hand.

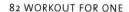

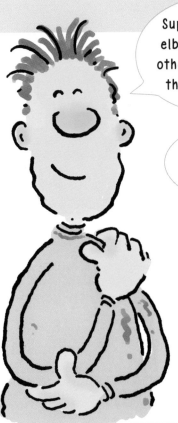

Supporting your elbow with your other hand, grasp the shoulder ...

... and squeeze the muscles firmly. Repeat on the other shoulder.

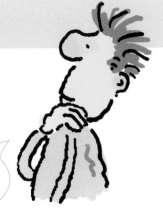

MOVE FIRST

Stiff shoulders and neck can restrict the blood circulation to and from your head, increasing the risk of headaches. Shoulders are more likely to become stiff when there are problems with the digestive system or when you are feeling depressed. Remember: prevention is better than cure.

NECK STRETCHES

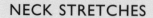

Repeat once

WHAT TO DO

Your neck muscles are the most used muscles in your body. Apart from when you are lying down, they constantly have to work to keep your head upright. If you have tried lifting someone's head you will know that it is the heaviest part of the body for its size.

Through over-use, it is common for neck muscles to get tired, leading to aches and restricted movement in the neck. These simple exercises are easy to do anywhere. In fact, I can do them while I am working at my computer. The more often you practise these stretches, the easier it will be to keep your neck in good shape.

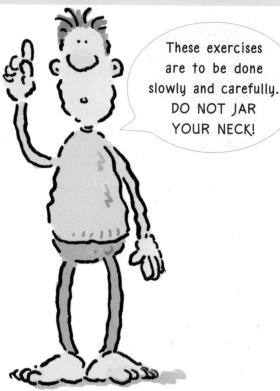

These exercises are to be done slowly and carefully. DO NOT JAR YOUR NECK!

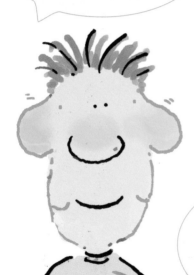

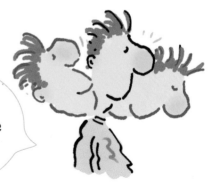

SHOULDER EXERCISES

WHAT TO DO

These two exercises are both excellent for keeping your chi moving through your shoulders.

Contract your muscles as far as you can as you lift your shoulders, filling yourself with air. On the outbreath you might find it a greater release to make a sound as you drop your shoulders. The rotations are helpful for maintaining the movement in your shoulders. This will reduce the risk of cartilage, tendons, ligaments and muscles tightening up.

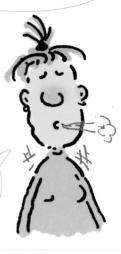

Breathing in, pull the shoulders as high as they will go ...

... and hold, keeping the shoulders tense.

Suddenly drop the shoulders as you breathe out. Repeat twice.

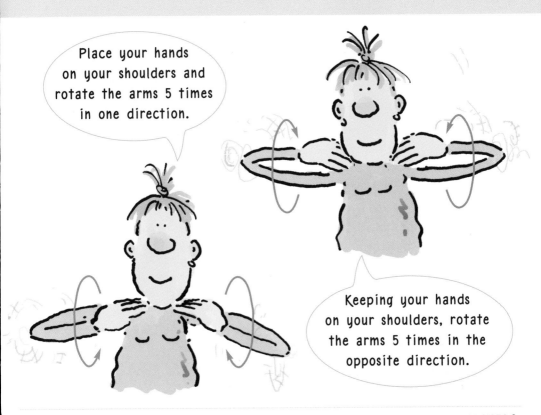

WHAT TO DO

You should be able to dispel a lot of the stored-up tension in your shoulders and upper back by pounding your shoulders. Ideal if you spend too much time at a computer or in a car, pounding your shoulders will greatly reduce the risk of building up lactic acids.

Hold the elbow of one arm with the hand of the other, so that you can stretch your arm across the front of your neck and reach behind the shoulder and neck. You should be able to pound your shoulder muscles quite vigorously. If they are sensitive to the touch, it might indicate that you need to eat more wholefoods and chew better.

HOW TO POUND

I find pounding with a loose fist the most versatile method. Keep the wrist loose and floppy, and give yourself as vigorous or as gentle a pounding as you like. For a more gentle pounding, try using the side or flat of your hand or the tips of your fingers. Each method creates a different sensation, so try them all out and choose one that suits you.

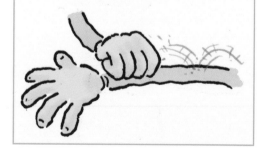

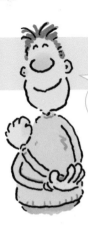

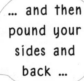

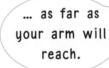

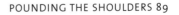

POUNDING THE ARMS

1 min

WHAT TO DO

Following each meridian line, pound up and down both arms, paying particular attention to any spots that are unusually sensitive. Such a spot may indicate an acupressure point that needs attention. I suggest that you go back to painful areas and spend a bit more time on them so that your chi flows more harmoniously.

Position the arm that you are pounding into a convenient place for each of the meridian lines to be pounded. Once you have pounded each meridian, you should be able to feel a warm buzz in your arms.

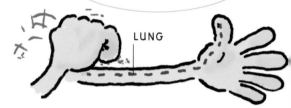

1. Pound down the inside of the arm, leading to the thumb.

LUNG

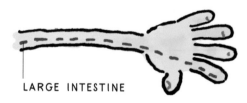

2. Turn the arm over and pound from the first finger to the shoulder.

LARGE INTESTINE

3. Turn the arm back. Pound down the middle of the arm to the second finger.

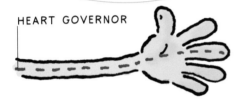

HEART GOVERNOR

5. Turn the arm back again and pound down the inside of the arm to the little finger.

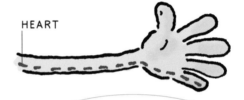

HEART

4. Turn the arm over. Pound up the middle of the arm to the shoulder.

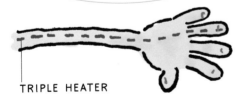

TRIPLE HEATER

6. Turn the arm over for the last time and pound up the outside from the little finger to the shoulder.

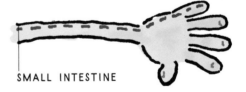

SMALL INTESTINE

All the meridians either run through, begin or end in your torso. In addition, there are two meridians – the conception and governing vessels – that only run through the centre of your back and front (see right).

The bladder meridian can be divided into a number of zones on your back, each relating to an internal organ. So, if you get a backache, it is a good idea to establish which zone it is in and then to check out the condition of the relevant organ. You can also work on the appropriate meridian to see if that helps relieve your backache.

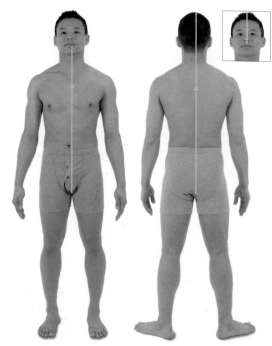

CONCEPTION VESSEL   GOVERNING VESSEL

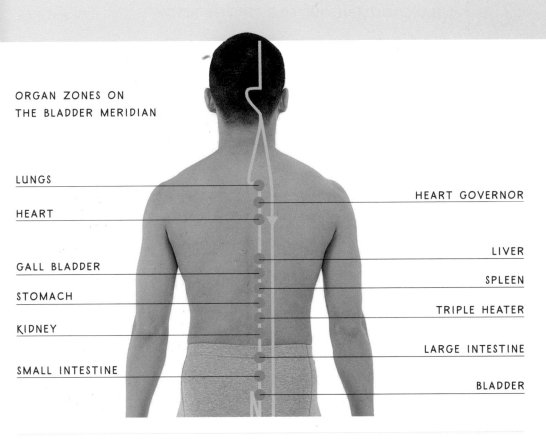

ORGAN ZONES ON
THE BLADDER MERIDIAN

LUNGS

HEART

GALL BLADDER

STOMACH

KIDNEY

SMALL INTESTINE

HEART GOVERNOR

LIVER

SPLEEN

TRIPLE HEATER

LARGE INTESTINE

BLADDER

POUNDING THE MIDDLE OF THE BODY

Repeat once

WHAT TO DO

The first of these exercises is not for the bus or train! Here is your chance to imitate Tarzan. Kneel down if you can. Then make a loud 'aaaaah' sound, so that your rib cage vibrates, giving your lungs an excellent internal massage. Pounding your chest at the same time will intensify the experience and really stir up the chi there as well as help you get rid of excess mucus.

Carry on pounding your lower back, then your buttocks. These are the biggest muscles you have, so there is plenty of blood and chi to get moving. Pound these muscles vigorously.

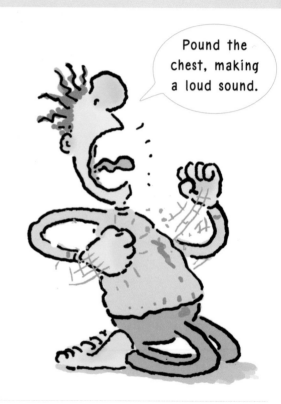

Pound the chest, making a loud sound.

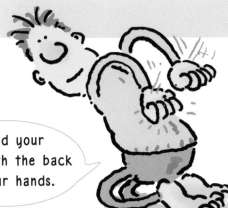

Kneel up and pound the hips and buttocks with a firm fist.

Pound your back with the back of your hands.

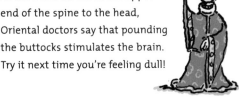

GIVE YOUR BRAIN A POUNDING

As the buttocks are at the opposite end of the spine to the head, Oriental doctors say that pounding the buttocks stimulates the brain. Try it next time you're feeling dull!

WHAT TO DO

This is a good time to jump up and loosen up a bit. Shaking is an excellent way to loosen up all your joints and increase your blood and lymph circulation. Try to get the shakes to start from your torso and spin out like a wave to your fingers and toes.

Feel free to jump around a bit and go a bit wild. It is good to try some spontaneous movements and let yourself go. Your body will naturally use this to make helpful adjustments to your chi. Make sure you have plenty of space so you do not feel confined or – worse – end up bumping into things.

> If you have been kneeling you may be feeling pain or pins and needles in the knees and ankles. Get up slowly!

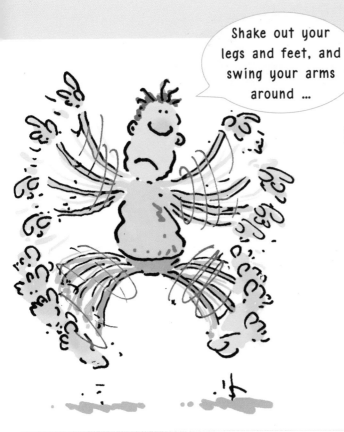
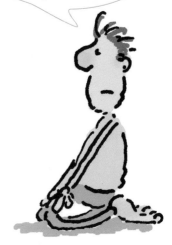

MASSAGING THE ABDOMEN

WHAT TO DO

The abdomen is unprotected by any bones and you may feel nervous about doing any kind of deep massage here. In fact, the organs at the front of your abdomen are flexible and respond well to massage, becoming toned up and more efficient.

These exercises show you how to get your fingers 'under your skin' so you can feel and work on the organs and deeper energies. Start gently and slowly and see how deep you can let your fingers sink into your abdomen. Stop massaging if you feel any pain.

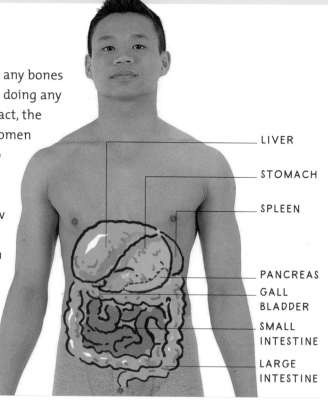

LIVER

STOMACH

SPLEEN

PANCREAS

GALL BLADDER

SMALL INTESTINE

LARGE INTESTINE

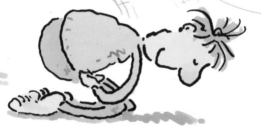

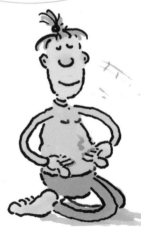

Kneel down and position your hands close together below your ribs. Breathe in and then ...

... breathe out as you bend down slowly, gently pushing your fingers up and under your ribs to the first finger joint.

Breathe in as you sit up again. This exercise massages the liver on the left and the stomach on the right.

ABDOMINAL MASSAGE – KNEELING 2

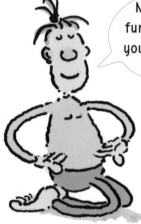

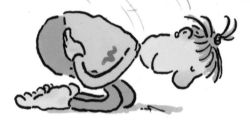

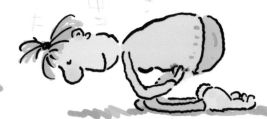

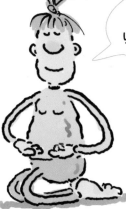

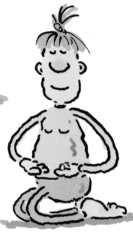

WHAT TO DO

You will find it easier to massage your abdomen if you lie down and raise your knees. This will relax your abdomen, making it easier to press into the soft tissue. As you work round in a clockwise direction, you will be following the path of your large intestine, helping to move your food along. This is a good massage to do if you suffer from constipation.

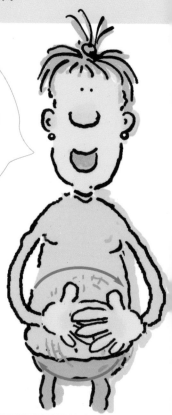

... and rub the abdomen in a clockwise direction, pressing firmly – this is the direction food passes through the large intestine.

Lie down on your back with your knees bent ...

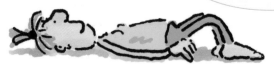

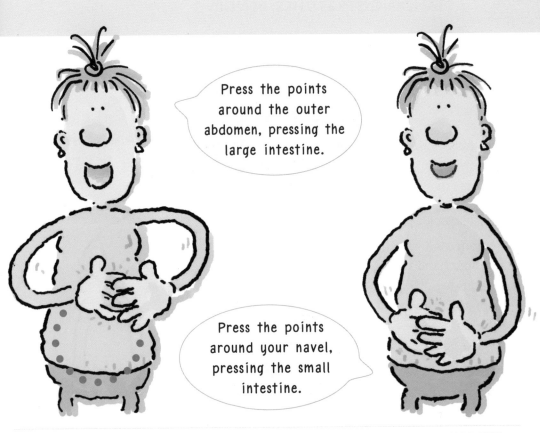

STANDING STRETCHES: BENDING

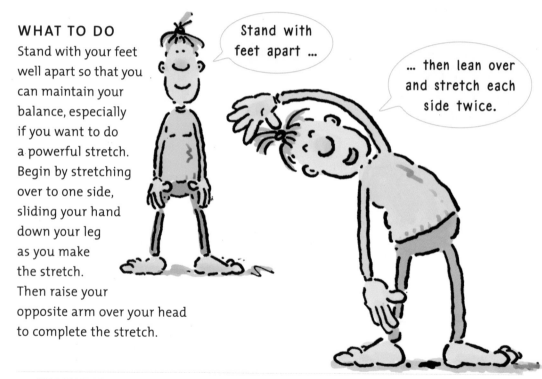

WHAT TO DO
Stand with your feet
well apart so that you
can maintain your
balance, especially
if you want to do
a powerful stretch.
Begin by stretching
over to one side,
sliding your hand
down your leg
as you make
the stretch.
Then raise your
opposite arm over your head
to complete the stretch.

Stand with
feet apart ...

... then lean over
and stretch each
side twice.

WHAT TO DO

As you twist your body, clasp your hands behind your neck to help add strength to the rotation of your upper body. If you feel any discomfort in your knees as you do this, try to twist your hips in the opposite direction to concentrate the stretch into your back.

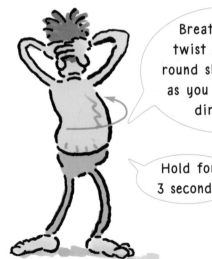

Breathing out, twist your body round slowly as far as you can in one direction.

Hold for 3 seconds.

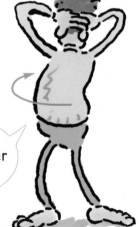

Repeat in the other direction.

WHAT TO DO

Stand, facing forwards, with your feet apart. Then turn to the side, turning your leading foot so your toes are pointing in the direction you are facing. Lean forwards, bending your knee. Place your hand over your leading knee to support it. Keep your body upright and stretch your trailing leg and hip. Practise this stretch, moving your feet further apart until you reach your natural limit.

> Stand with your feet apart and turn to face one side.

> Lunge, stretching the inside of each leg 3 times.

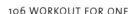

WHAT TO DO

Stand with your feet wide apart. Bending one knee, while keeping the other leg straight, lower your body to the floor, stretching to one side. Place your hands on the floor for support as you try to lower yourself as far as you can.

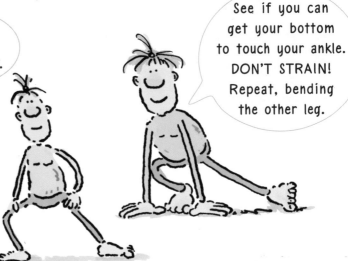

Stand with feet wide apart.

Bend one knee and begin to lower yourself downwards.

See if you can get your bottom to touch your ankle. DON'T STRAIN! Repeat, bending the other leg.

WHAT TO DO

This is a huge stretch for the front of your body, particularly the front of your upper legs. You may need to ease into it over several weeks. Start slowly with some firm cushions for support, using your elbows to gently lower yourself down. If at any time you feel unstable, or the stretch is too strong, stop and move onto the next page. Once you are in the full stretch position, raise your arms above your head and you will feel a powerful stretch from your chest to your knees.

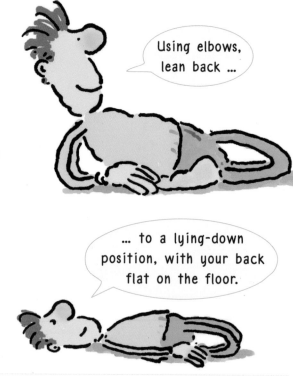

Using elbows, lean back ...

... to a lying-down position, with your back flat on the floor.

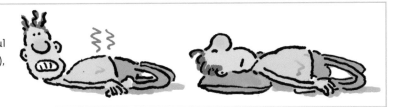

Stretch your arms out and hold the position for 10 seconds.

Don't forget to breathe!

Come up slowly, using your elbows, and stretch forwards.

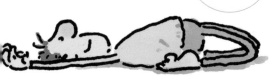

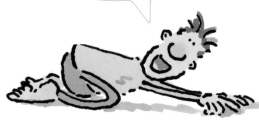

WHAT TO DO

Sit with your legs straight in front of you and as far apart as possible. Over the next few weeks, increase the distance apart you set your legs, to gradually increase the stretch. Stretch forward, holding your leg. Grab your toes and pull them back towards your head.

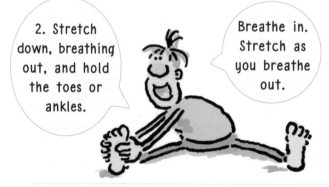

1. Stretch your legs as wide apart as possible ...

... toes pointing towards the head.

2. Stretch down, breathing out, and hold the toes or ankles.

Breathe in. Stretch as you breathe out.

3. Repeat on the other leg.

WHAT TO DO

This twisting stretch is excellent for loosening up your lower back. You may even feel a click as one of your vertebrae re-aligns itself.

Crossing your legs will make the stretch more effective and you can use your legs to push yourself round. Stretch slowly and try to avoid making any sudden movements.

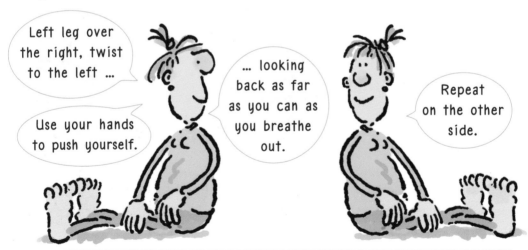

Left leg over the right, twist to the left ...

Use your hands to push yourself.

... looking back as far as you can as you breathe out.

Repeat on the other side.

SITTING STRETCHES: INSIDE LEG

WHAT TO DO

Most children can push their knees down to the ground while sitting. As adults we lose this flexibility but this exercise can help us to regain it!

Sit on the floor so that the soles of your feet are touching each other and your heels are as close to your body as possible. Let your knees drop out to the sides. Hold your feet with your hands and put your elbows against the inside of your knees. As you breathe out, lean forward as far as possible while pushing your knees towards the ground with your elbows.

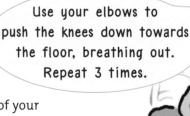

WHAT TO DO

This exercise is good for your lower back and your spine as you roll on each vertebra. Sit on a soft floor with plenty of space behind you, and cross your legs.

Hold your feet in your hands and roll backwards. Keep your back curved and roll all the way to the back of your head and back up to sitting. Soon you will be able to roll back and forth easily.

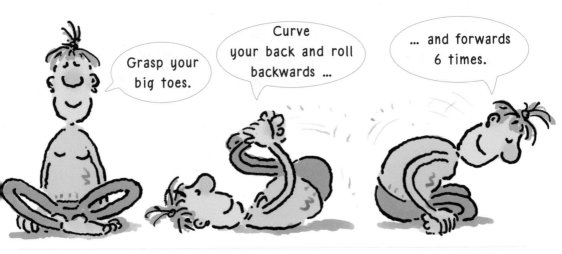

Grasp your big toes.

Curve your back and roll backwards ...

... and forwards 6 times.

WHAT TO DO

Lying on your back and drawing your knees to your chest helps tighten your abdominal muscles and stretch your lower back. Swinging your knees from side to side rotates and stretches your lower back.

To stretch out your shoulders, try the 'cat' stretch. Stretch an arm out in front and pull slowly, getting your chest as close to the floor as you can.

Next, to stretch the lower back, push up your upper body, straightening your arms slightly, and let your abdomen sag down .

LYING STRETCHES: OPENING

PRESSING AND RUBBING LEG AND FOOT POINTS

There are six meridians running up and down each leg. Three of them – spleen, liver and kidney – run up the insides of your legs, and three – bladder, gall bladder and stomach – flow down the backs and outsides of your legs. All begin or end at your toes except the kidney meridian, which ends at the sole of the foot.

All these meridians continue from the top of your legs up your body. The longest meridians – bladder, gall bladder and stomach – stretch all the way from your head to your toes. This is why massaging your feet can reduce headaches.

Working on any of these meridian lines increases your connection with the ground and helps increase the movement of chi vertically through your body.

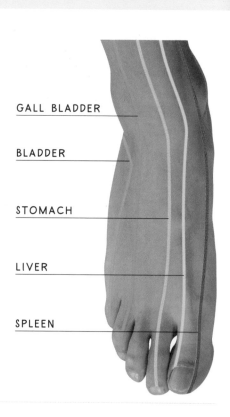

GALL BLADDER

BLADDER

STOMACH

LIVER

SPLEEN

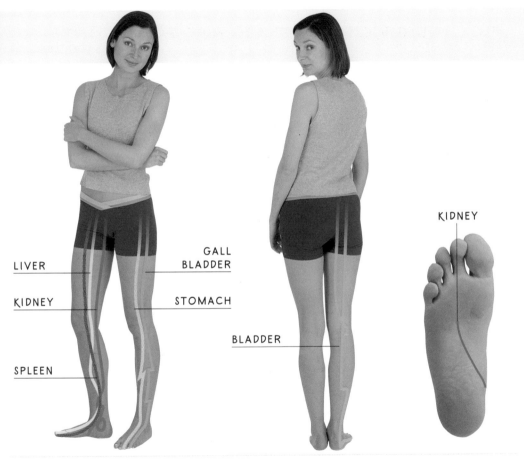

LIVER

KIDNEY

SPLEEN

GALL
BLADDER

STOMACH

BLADDER

KIDNEY

POUNDING THE LEGS

WHAT TO DO

You can pound your legs in a standing or sitting position. Just as you did when pounding the arms (see page 90), follow the path of each leg meridian. Pound firmly all the way up and down, using both hands.

You can make the backs of your legs softer and easier to pound if you bend your knees slightly and point your toes away from you. Use a loose fist and flexible wrist. When you have pounded each meridian on one leg, repeat the sequence on the other one.

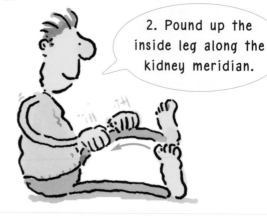

1. Starting at the buttocks, beat with both fists down the back of the leg to the foot along the bladder meridian.

2. Pound up the inside leg along the kidney meridian.

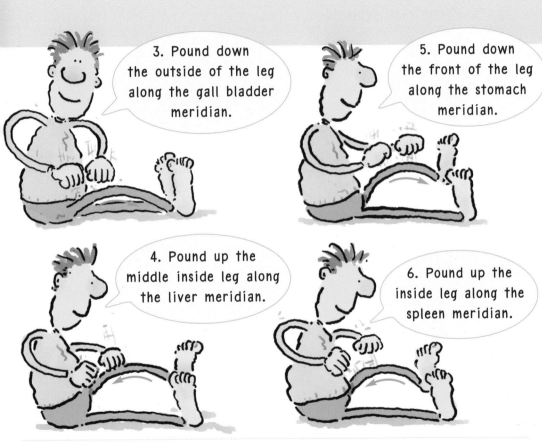

WHAT TO DO

One of the challenges of working on these points is finding a convenient position for your legs and feet that allows you to reach the points comfortably. Sitting on the floor makes it easier. Bend one leg over the other to reach the lower leg and foot points.

As usual, the more you practise, the quicker you will become at finding the points and being able to home in on the exact spots.

Find the location.

Rub the point as you breathe in.

Press the point for 5 seconds as you breathe out.

WALKING BAREFOOT

Try massaging your feet by walking barefoot on different surfaces. Grass, sand and pebbles will all massage the bottoms of your feet and stimulate the acupressure points there, encouraging your chi to flow more strongly.

Try this exercise in the morning if you want to energize your chi, and in the evening to settle it.

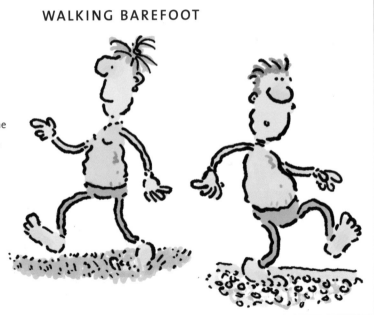

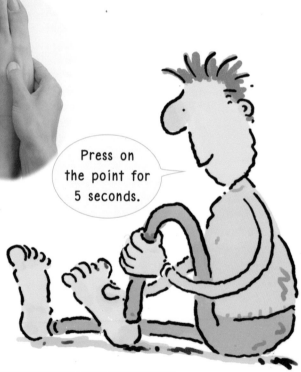

WHAT TO DO

Pressing this point will re-energize you if you're feeling lethargic. Sit with one knee bent. Find the groove between the bones that lead to your big toe and second toe. Starting from the web at the foot of your toes, slide your thumb back about four finger-widths towards your ankle until you get close to the end of the groove. This is the acupressure point. To help release chi, press firmly and slide your thumb down the groove towards your toes with a strong out-breath. Repeat on the other foot.

Press on the point for 5 seconds.

GOOD FOR

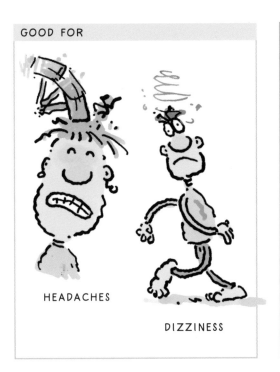

HEADACHES

DIZZINESS

LIVER MERIDIAN (yin)

Good for increasing activity and the ability to get things done, this meridian line is also often associated with impatience and anger when overactive.

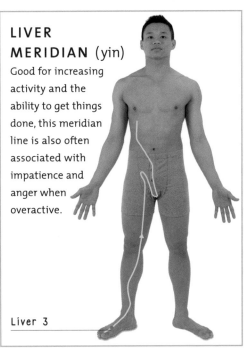

Liver 3

GUSHING SPRING
Kidney meridian point 1

Repeat 3 times on each foot

WHAT TO DO

This is a good pressure point to work on if you're lacking in confidence or energy.

Sit with one leg folded over the other, and bend the foot slightly with your hands. From the side you will see a strong crease running along the centre. Press into this crease deeply, rubbing your thumb along it from the heel towards the middle toe. At the base of the ball of your foot, you should feel a bone. Press deeply into your foot here: you should feel a dull ache. Breathe chi into this point as far as you can. Repeat on the other foot.

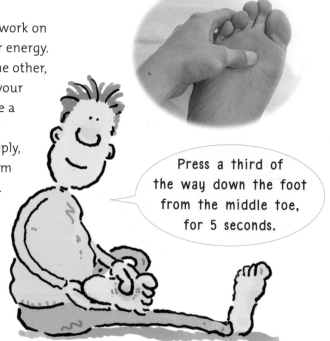

Press a third of the way down the foot from the middle toe, for 5 seconds.

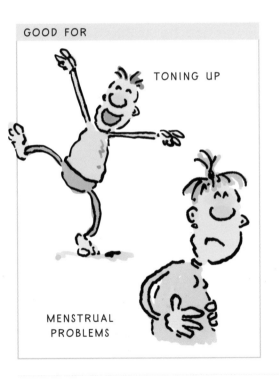

TONING UP

MENSTRUAL
PROBLEMS

KIDNEY MERIDIAN (yang)

Responsible for blood quality, fluid balance and elimination of waste from the blood, this meridian is good for confidence, vitality and the health of reproductive organs. An imbalance in chi flow here can create feelings of fear and anxiety.

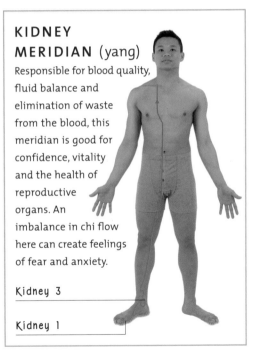

Kidney 3

Kidney 1

GREAT GROOVE
Kidney meridian point 3

Repeat 3 times on each leg

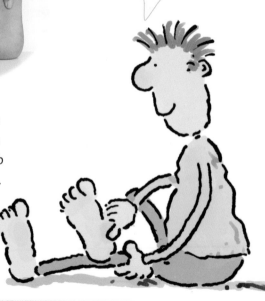

Press half-way between the tip of the ankle bone and the Achilles tendon for 5 seconds.

WHAT TO DO

Work on this point to relieve backache and menstrual pains. Rest your foot on your other leg so that you can see the inside of your ankle. Feel around the back of your inner ankle bone until you find a groove between the bone and the Achilles tendon. Slide your thumb up and down until you find the exact spot. Grip the outside of your leg with your fingers to make it easy to apply pressure into this acupressure point. Keep working the point until it has warmed up. Repeat on the other foot.

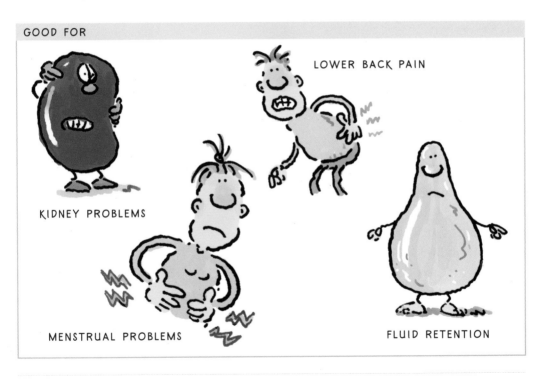

GOOD FOR

KIDNEY PROBLEMS

LOWER BACK PAIN

MENSTRUAL PROBLEMS

FLUID RETENTION

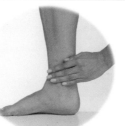 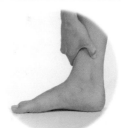

MEETING PLACE OF 3 YIN MERIDIANS
Spleen meridian point 6

Repeat 3 times
on each leg

WHAT TO DO

The chi in this meridian helps prevent mood swings. Place your little finger just on your inside ankle bone. Your index finger should fall just behind your shin bone – this is where the point lies. Slide your thumb up and down the rear of the bone until you find a spot that produces a sharp pain. Press into this point slowly and focus on moving chi energy up your legs.

> Place hand on leg, little finger above ankle bone – the point is where the index finger falls.

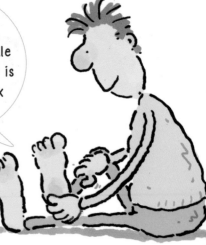

---
*AVOID IF PREGNANT

GOOD FOR

ANY PROBLEMS RELATING TO REPRODUCTIVE ORGANS

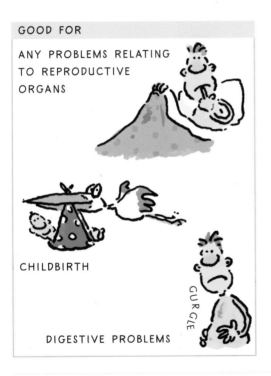

CHILDBIRTH

DIGESTIVE PROBLEMS

GURGLE

SPLEEN MERIDIAN (yin)

This meridian is responsible for cleanliness, order, stability and decisiveness. When the chi here is out of balance, it can cause mood swings, self-pity and lack of direction.

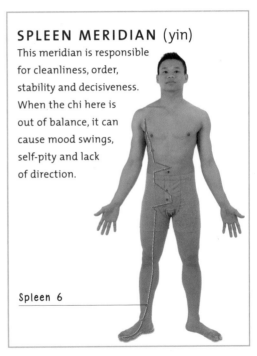

Spleen 6

IN THE MOUNTAIN
Bladder meridian point 57

Repeat 3 times on each leg

WHAT TO DO

If you're feeling insecure about the past, you may find it helpful to work on this point. Sit with one knee bent. Slide your thumb down the back of your calf muscle, looking for a shallow groove that runs down the centre from the thickest point. Run your thumb to the top of the groove about one third of the way down from the back of the knee. Press into the muscle until you find a sensitive area – this is the point. Press into it to activate the chi. Repeat on the other leg.

> Press in the top of the groove at the beginning of the calf muscle for 5 seconds.

GOOD FOR

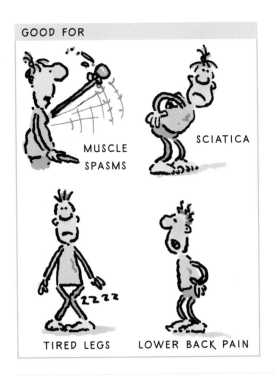

MUSCLE SPASMS

SCIATICA

TIRED LEGS

LOWER BACK PAIN

BLADDER MERIDIAN (yang)

This meridian is responsible for memory and the quality of body fluids, which make up 70 per cent of your body. An imbalance causes insecurities about the past.

Bladder 57

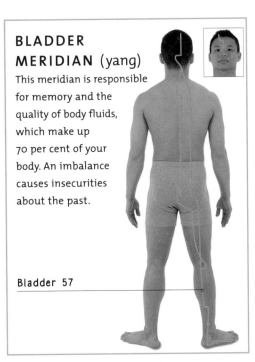

LIFE TOMB SPRING
Gall bladder meridian point 34

Repeat 3 times on each leg

WHAT TO DO

Try working on this point if you're feeling tense and irritable. Sit so that your leg is bent at an angle of 90 degrees, and find the bottom of your knee cap. Now move your finger to the outside of the leg until you locate a bony indentation. Press into the hollow with your thumb and direct your force downwards slightly, against the ridge of the bone. You may need to open your leg slightly to get into the point. Imagine you are breathing chi right into your knee as you work this point. Repeat on the other knee.

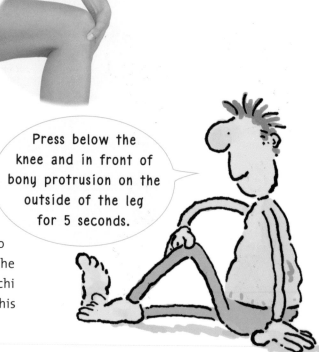

Press below the knee and in front of bony protrusion on the outside of the leg for 5 seconds.

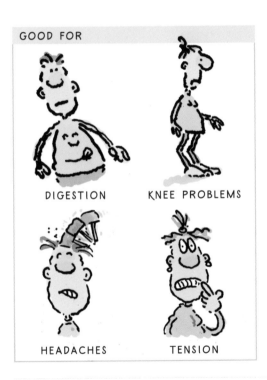

GOOD FOR

DIGESTION

KNEE PROBLEMS

HEADACHES

TENSION

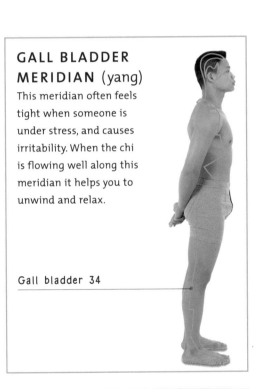

GALL BLADDER MERIDIAN (yang)

This meridian often feels tight when someone is under stress, and causes irritability. When the chi is flowing well along this meridian it helps you to unwind and relax.

Gall bladder 34

3-MILE POINT
Stomach meridian point 36

Repeat 3 times on each leg

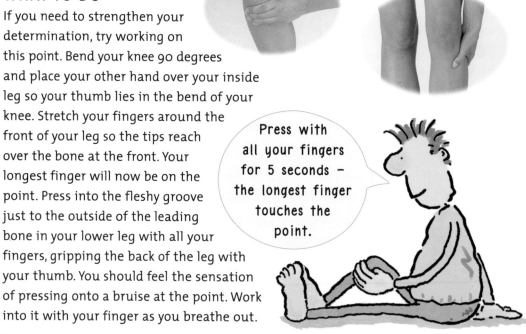

WHAT TO DO

If you need to strengthen your determination, try working on this point. Bend your knee 90 degrees and place your other hand over your inside leg so your thumb lies in the bend of your knee. Stretch your fingers around the front of your leg so the tips reach over the bone at the front. Your longest finger will now be on the point. Press into the fleshy groove just to the outside of the leading bone in your lower leg with all your fingers, gripping the back of the leg with your thumb. You should feel the sensation of pressing onto a bruise at the point. Work into it with your finger as you breathe out.

Press with all your fingers for 5 seconds – the longest finger touches the point.

GOOD FOR

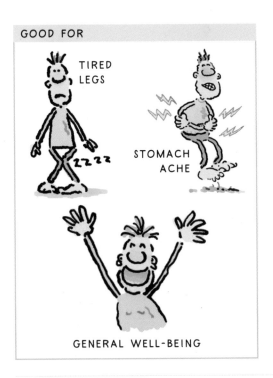

TIRED LEGS

STOMACH ACHE

GENERAL WELL-BEING

STOMACH MERIDIAN (yang)

When flowing well, stomach energy is associated with strength, determination and moving forwards.

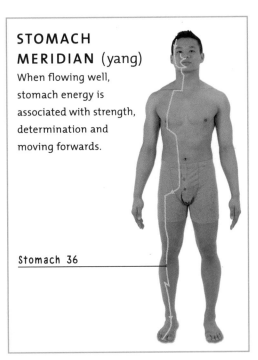

Stomach 36

KNEE AND HIP ROTATION

WHAT TO DO

Your knees are primarily designed to bend in one direction – back and forth – but it is helpful to increase mobility in your knee joints. For the knee rotation exercise (right), support your knees with your hands and keep your feet together so that your knees rotate together, supporting each other. Do not force your knees – simply let them take up the free circular movement.

Use the hip rotation exercise (far right) to stretch out your lower back and increase mobility. Start by doing this exercise slowly, and then increase the speed a little to get some motion into the movement.

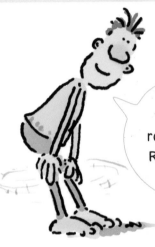

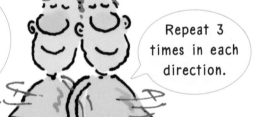

WHAT TO DO

The physical pressure felt by your ankles, combined with their narrow shape, makes it easy for your chi to get compressed and stuck in them. After a long day, you should find that relieving pressure here and allowing your chi energy to flow freely allows your chi to disperse, leaving you with a wonderful feeling of lightness.

Doing these exercises regularly on both feet will help prevent a build-up of chi in your feet and ankles.

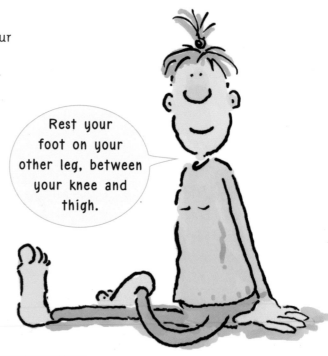

Rest your foot on your other leg, between your knee and thigh.

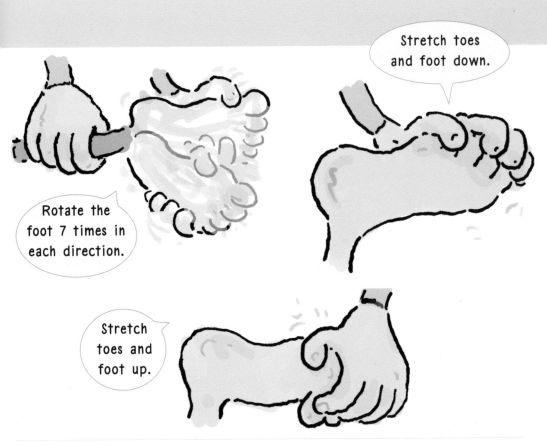

TOE WORKOUT

Repeat once on other foot

WHAT TO DO

The idea here is to get your chi moving from the tips of your toes all the way along your meridians to the top of your head and out. Because your feet can spend so much time confined to your shoes, it is important to give your toes a good stretch and massage to open up the chi again.

There are acupressure points at the sides of the base of your toenails. Give them a good squeeze before you pull your finger away from your toe to extend your energy.

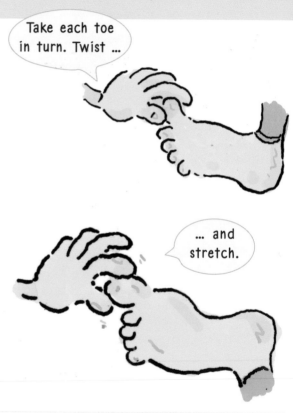

Take each toe in turn. Twist ...

... and stretch.

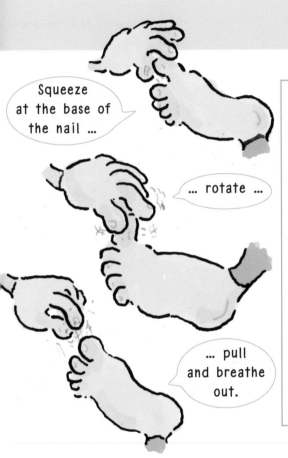

Squeeze at the base of the nail ...

... rotate ...

... pull and breathe out.

GENERATING CHI

To extend your chi energy in your toes, hold the base of each toe in turn between your thumb and forefinger. Pull your finger and thumb away from the first toe smartly as though you are creating a little spark as they leave. Breathe out quickly at the same time and imagine you are feeding the tip of your toe with energy, so that the spark starts a flame. As you pull your finger and thumb away, extend the flame as far as you can.

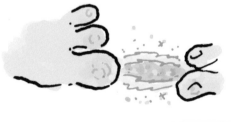

LAST FOOT WORKOUT

Repeat once on other foot

WHAT TO DO

To finish working on your feet, first massage all around each ankle with the fingers and thumb of one hand. Work into all the indentations and areas that chi can get stuck. Move your ankle to help open areas to press into.

Next, slide your thumbs along the grooves on the top of your feet pushing chi towards your toes. Feel for any sensitive spots that might need extra attention.

Lastly, pound the bottoms of your feet with a loose fist to stimulate the chi there.

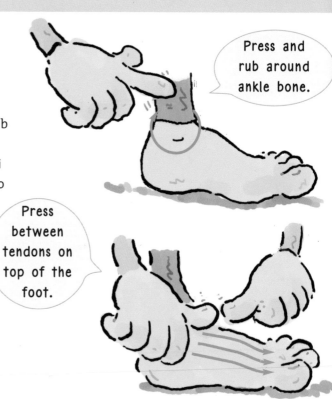

Press and rub around ankle bone.

Press between tendons on top of the foot.

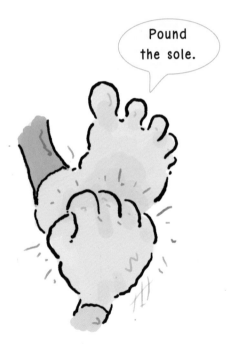

SOAKING YOUR FEET

When you want to draw chi down from your mind, to calm down or to sleep well, try soaking your feet and ankles in hot, salty water. This is an excellent way to relax at the end of the day .

WHAT TO DO

To complete your workout, jump up and shake yourself off so that your energy finds its own harmony again. Feel free to go wild and loosen all your limbs. If you have any music that really gets you going, now is the time to put it on.

Finally, relax and repeat the Tuning In exercise (pages 16–21) to see what changes you notice.

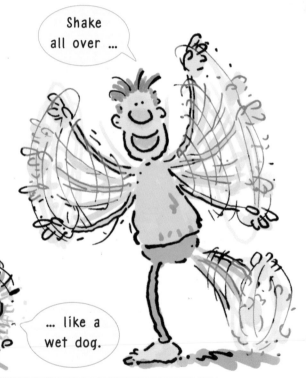

Shake all over ...

... like a wet dog.

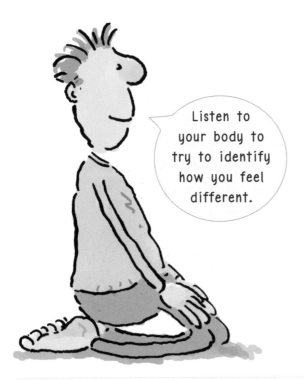

Listen to your body to try to identify how you feel different.

WORKOUT FOR TWO

If there are two of you, why not try the Workout for Two exercises, which start on page 158.

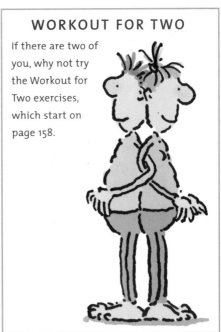

PROGRAMMES

This section features three different workout routines, with different objectives and requiring different amounts of time to complete. Each is presented as a sequence of quick visual reminders to each of the exercises. If you forget the steps or technique involved, refer to the page number next to the image and read through the exercise in full.

The first programme contains all the exercises and acupressure work included in the previous section in the order that it appears there. It will take about 45 minutes to complete. The other two programmes are shorter. The 25-minute routine is designed as an ideal wake-up call. The final programme takes just 10 minutes to complete and contains all the exercises you can do on a bus or train, or in an office, without attracting too much attention.

Of course, you can make up your own programmes too. For example, to unwind at the end of the day you might simply choose to do all the stretches in the book. Tailor your routine to suit your own needs and situation.

WHAT TO DO

Sometimes it's hard to get going on this routine, but usually, after the first few minutes, everything starts to flow naturally. Don't worry about how you feel before you start – dive in and enjoy it.

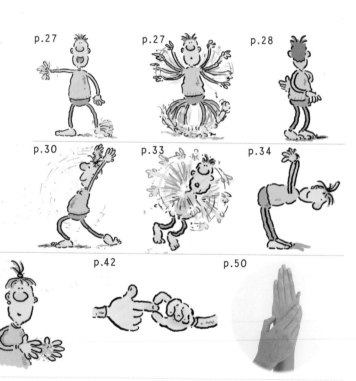

p.27

p.27

p.28

p.30

p.33

p.34

p.37

p.40

p.42

p.50

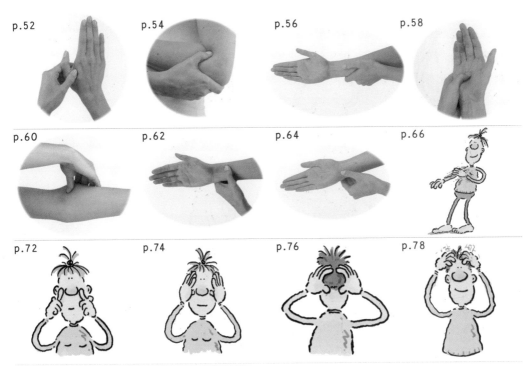

p.52 p.54 p.56 p.58

p.60 p.62 p.64 p.66

p.72 p.74 p.76 p.78

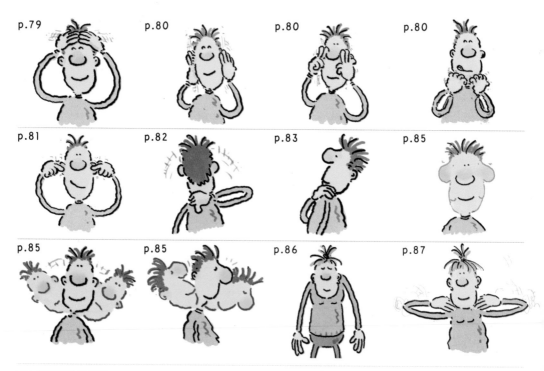

p.79   p.80   p.80   p.80

p.81   p.82   p.83   p.85

p.85   p.85   p.86   p.87

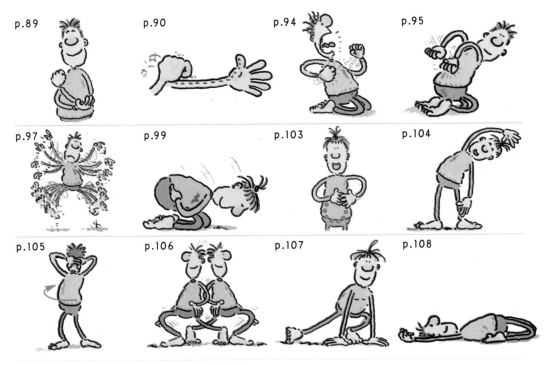

p.89

p.90

p.94

p.95

p.97

p.99

p.103

p.104

p.105

p.106

p.107

p.108

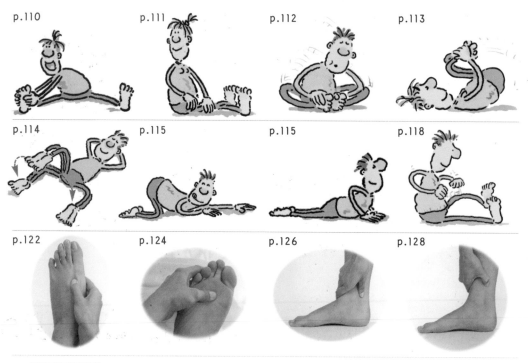

p.110   p.111   p.112   p.113

p.114   p.115   p.115   p.118

p.122   p.124   p.126   p.128

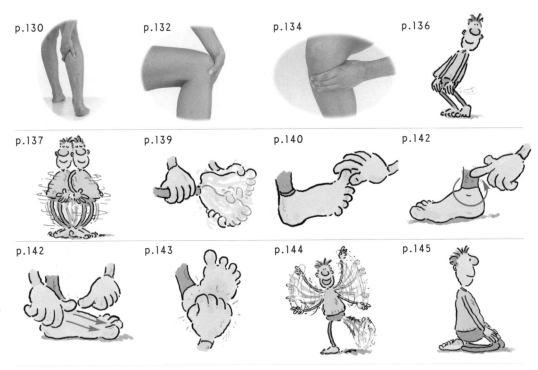

p.130

p.132

p.134

p.136

p.137

p.139

p.140

p.142

p.142

p.143

p.144

p.145

PROGRAMME 2

WHAT TO DO

Use this routine when you want to get your chi moving but are short of time. I have focused on the more active and dynamic exercises. After a couple of run-throughs, you will be able to fall out of bed and straight into this routine.

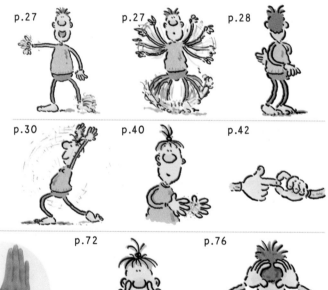

p.27   p.27   p.28

p.30   p.40   p.42

p.50

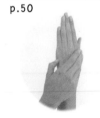

p.52

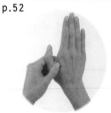

p.72

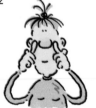

p.76

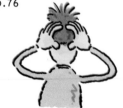

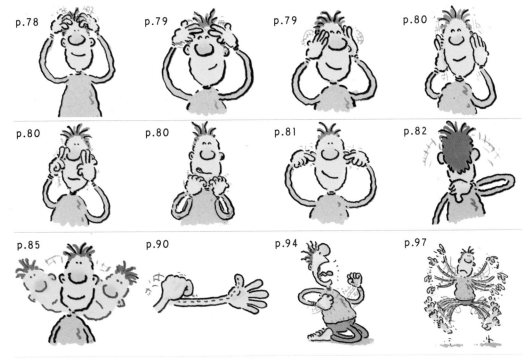

p.78

p.79

p.79

p.80

p.80

p.80

p.81

p.82

p.85

p.90

p.94

p.97

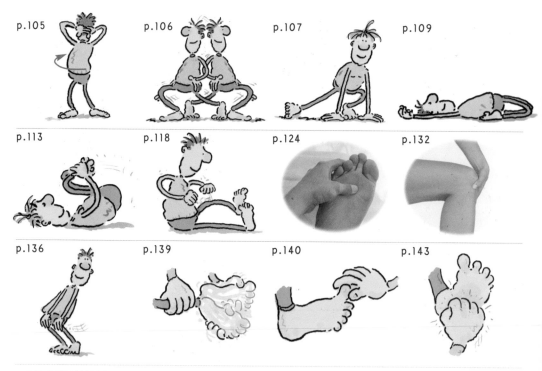

p.105

p.106

p.107

p.109

p.113

p.118

p.124

p.132

p.136

p.139

p.140

p.143

PROGRAMME 3

WHAT TO DO

This routine is around 10 minutes of bliss, and can be done wherever you are. It is essential if you work at a computer.

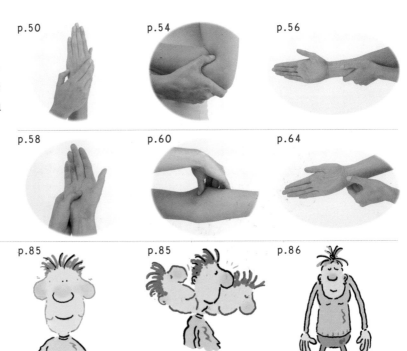

p.50   p.54   p.56

p.58   p.60   p.64

p.83   p.85   p.85   p.86

WORKOUT FOR TWO

The idea that two people can together achieve more than their individual efforts combined is certainly true of exercise. With these exercises for two you will be able to stretch and move one another's chi energy in ways you could only dream of on your own.

By exercising with another person you also develop your ability to interact constructively and to communicate through touch. If one picture is worth a thousand words, an affectionate hug or squeeze is worth ten thousand.

This is where you learn to give and take, when to yield, and when to be strong and supportive. Whenever you are working with someone else it is essential that you do everything slowly, so that both of you can relax and develop mutual trust. Do not be afraid to expose your weaknesses and ask for help. And be careful and considerate in finding out what is appropriate for your exercise partner.

SHIATSU MASSAGE

Shiatsu is quite simply Do In exercises done by one person to another. One person relaxes while the other rubs, pounds, presses, stretches and massages the other's body. This form of shiatsu is excellent for helping you stay relaxed, supple and full of energy. It is also a great way to communicate.

WALK, I said!!!

Another's touch can convey love, healing or comfort. You naturally put your hand to any part of the body where you feel pain. In this way, a dialogue develops to produce a powerful therapy.

Shiatsu practitioner Wataru Ohashi tells a story set in the Orient of a young, newly married woman whose life was made miserable by the abnormally cruel nature of her husband's mother. After many years of hardship, she decided the only way to save her family was to poison her mother-in-law. A herbalist gave her a potion and instructed her to combine it with a shiatsu every day for three months.

Within two months, the young woman began to understand why her mother-in-law behaved as she did. Through the shiatsu she could feel what her weaknesses and insecurities were. At the same time, her mother-in-law became more relaxed and appreciative of her daily shiatsu and began to grow fond of her daughter-in-law.

The young woman realized she was making a terrible mistake and rushed back to the herbalist for an antidote. The herbalist smiled and admitted that the potion was, in fact, a harmless flower water. She had known that regular shiatsu would help to resolve the differences between them.

SHIATSU IN PRACTICE

I have worked as a shiatsu therapist and teacher for more than twenty years and in that time I have learned what works. The reality is that some people respond well to shiatsu and have incredible results, while others experience slower benefits even though their complaints may be easier to treat. Most people come for stress relief, aches and pains (often in the back and neck), PMT, lack of energy and stress-related problems, such as allergies and skin problems.

Shiatsu has to be experienced to be appreciated. On the following pages you will find a simple shiatsu routine for the back which you can try with a friend.

STRETCHING LOWER BACK AND INSIDE LEGS

WHAT TO DO

Sit facing each other with your legs apart and feet touching. If one of you is considerably taller than the other, let the shorter person put their feet against the other's inner leg.

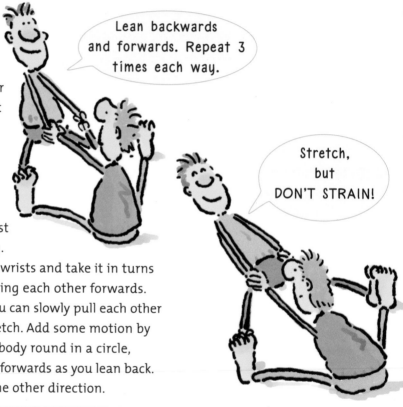

Lean backwards and forwards. Repeat 3 times each way.

Stretch, but DON'T STRAIN!

Hold each other's wrists and take it in turns to lean back, stretching each other forwards. Work together, so you can slowly pull each other to the optimum stretch. Add some motion by moving your upper body round in a circle, stretching the other forwards as you lean back. Repeat, circling in the other direction.

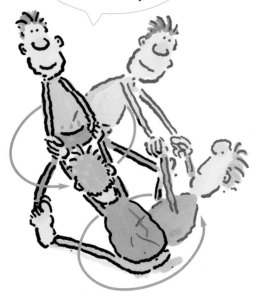

WORKING TOGETHER

If you are finding it difficult to relate to someone close to you, exercising together may bring you closer. Forget any problem issues between you and focus on making the exercises work for you both.

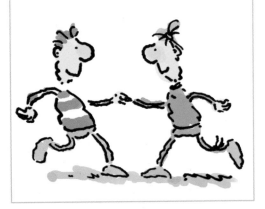

STRETCHING CALF MUSCLES

WHAT TO DO

Kneel by the side of your friend, who is lying on their back. Lift one leg and let it rest on your shoulder. Put one foot forward so you can lean onto it to make the stretch. Support the lifted leg with one arm close to the knee while holding the other leg onto the floor with your other hand. Now lean forward to make the stretch. Repeat with the other leg before swapping over.

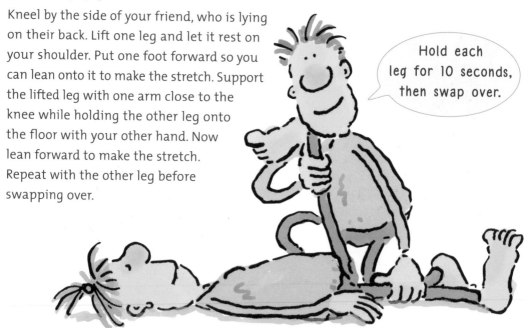

Hold each leg for 10 seconds, then swap over.

STRETCHING LOWER BACK

WHAT TO DO

Do not attempt this exercise if either of you have a history of back injuries or a stiff or painful back.

Sit back to back, one person with their legs out straight and the other with folded knees. Lock your elbows together. If you are the person with the bent knees, push up, while your friend leans forwards until you are lying on top of your friend. Try to relax, while your friend releases tension from the legs and back.

Point your toes towards your head.

Relax!

Lean forward as your friend pushes up. Hold for 15 seconds. Swap over.

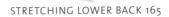

BACK STRETCHING

WHAT TO DO

It can feel weird being stretched over someone's back, so doing this exercise requires a strong degree of trust. It is essential for the person being stretched to relax as, if they tighten up, they may fall off. When you both feel confident, the supporting partner can bounce gently to loosen up the other.

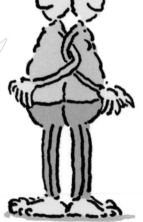

Stand back to back and link elbows.

> ### WARNING!
> **Avoid this exercise if you have a history of back problems.**
>
> Make sure your partner is of a similar weight and height and that the space you are exercising in is clear of furniture.

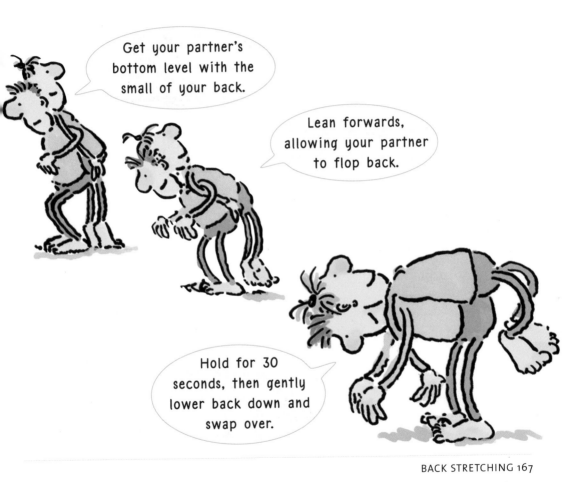

POUNDING

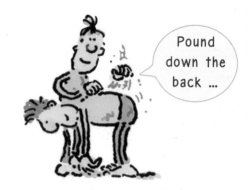

WHAT TO DO

Pounding will loosen up your body and get your chi flowing. Try to get your friend into a comfortable position in which it is easy for you to pound them. They could be lying down, sitting on a stool, standing or bending over.

LOOSE WRISTS

Try to put your hands into relaxed fists and keep your wrists loose so the pounding motion comes from your elbow. Work with your friend to find the ideal intensity.

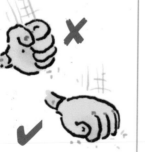

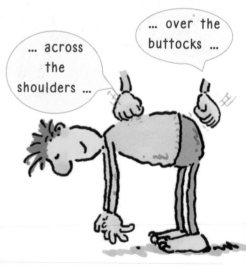

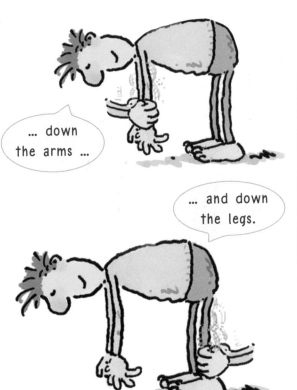

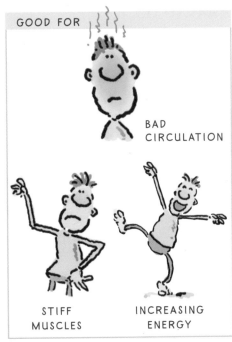

BRUSHING

WHAT TO DO

Brushing helps move and clear your superficial chi, encouraging fresh chi to come back into your body.

Brush your hands smartly across your friend's clothes or skin, while breathing out strongly. Work around your friend's body slowly, starting with their back and working out to the limbs.

Experiment with the type of touch you apply. Try making contact using your fingertips and then with the palms of your hands. Keep your wrists and hands as loose as possible, so the brushing movement is driven from your shoulders and elbows.

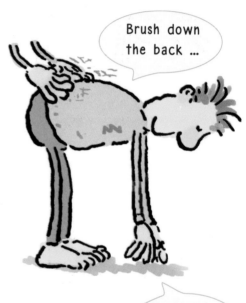

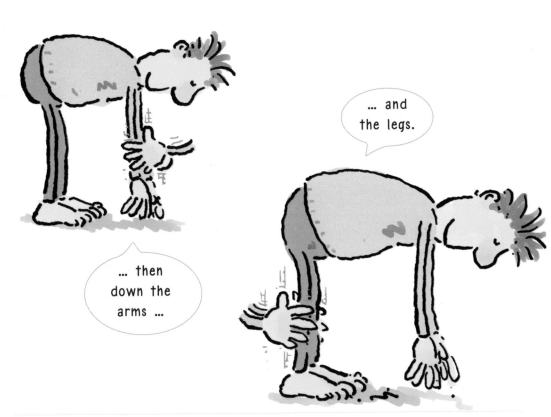

ROCKING

WHAT TO DO

With your friend lying on their front, hold the hips and rock them from side to side. You should be able to rock the whole body from here, so your friend's head and feet should move slightly as you rock the hips. Watch their back carefully to see if the spine moves smoothly. Any stiff areas will need attention.

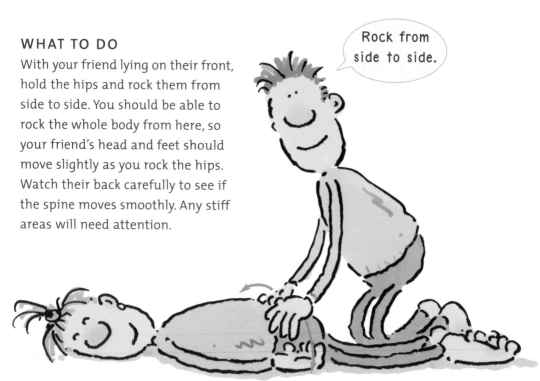

90 secs

FINGER PRESSURE

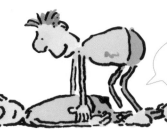

Stand astride the body.

WHAT TO DO

Stand astride your friend's prone body and place your fingers either side of the spine. Rub up and down the muscles of the back by sliding the skin over the muscles rather than sliding your fingers over the skin.

Talk with your friend to find out how much pressure is appropriate. Slowly work down the back to the buttocks.

Make small, circular movements. Move the skin over the muscles below.

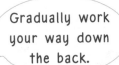

Gradually work your way down the back.

HAND PRESSURE

WHAT TO DO

Still standing astride your friend, push down on their back with open hands, starting at the top of the back. Work together, breathing out each time you press down. Ask your friend to breathe into the area of your hands before you push, so that you can maximize the movement as you lean onto your palms. Work all the way down to the feet, taking care to avoid pressing on the backs of the knees.

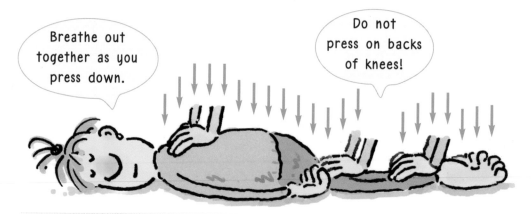

FOOT PRESSURE

WHAT TO DO

This is ideal for relieving mental tension and stress. A good way to massage someone else's feet is to use your own. With your friend lying face down, turn their feet, so that the toes point inwards. Stand with your back to your friend with your toes pointing out. Keep your weight on the balls of your feet and press onto the soles of your friend's feet with your heels. You may find it helpful to hold onto a chair for balance. Now swap over and go back to page 168, so you both get to feel good.

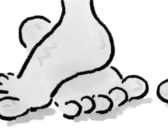

Point your friend's toes inwards ...

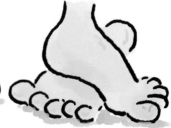

... and put your heels GENTLY on their arches.

Imagine you are gently treading grapes.

NOW
FIND OUT
MORE

Now that you have completed all the hard work, sit back and read more about the theory behind the practice. This section explains in more detail the nature of chi energy and how it works so that you can appreciate the key role of the meridians and acupressure points when you exercise.

The principles of yin and yang are also explained, revealing a whole new way of understanding the world around you. This will enable you to make connections between how you feel and your surroundings or situation, and allow you to harness the positive – and negative – forces around you to enhance your life.

Finally, a section outlining the theory of macrobiotics and its link with the principles of yin and yang and with the Do In exercises in this book reveals how to give your health an extra boost.

CHI ENERGY

For 3,000 years there has been a widespread belief in a living energy that flows throughout nature and is the essence of everything. The most complete records concerning this energy are found in the East: in China it is called 'chi'; in India it is called 'prana'; and in Japan it is called 'ki'. Chi is the flow of electromagnetic energy and, in a human being, it flows all around the body along invisible pathways known as meridians.

CHI'S UNIVERSAL PRESENCE

Throughout the universe, each object takes in and gives out chi. The larger an object, the greater its potential for moving chi. This makes the earth, moon, sun and other planets and galaxies important in terms of chi. Not only does the earth continually give out chi, which we experience as rising energy, but it also receives chi from all the other planets, which we experience as descending energy.

This movement of energy is all around us. The more natural your environment, the more freely chi will flow. Consequently, you will find that you have more energy walking through the countryside than in a large, modern, indoor shopping centre. A building made of organic materials is more relaxing and less tiring than one made of, and furnished with, synthetic materials that carry their own static charge. This also applies to clothing.

CHI WITHIN THE BODY

Chi energy is both influenced by, and will influence, a physical structure. One way of looking at this is to consider the action of water on a rough terrain of mud, sand and stones. As the water passes over the rough terrain, it flows along the natural valleys, skirting the sandbanks and swirling in the rockpools. Over the course of time, the flow of the water itself changes the terrain, creating deep-cut rivers, wider pools and new islands.

Now take the analogy a little further. Imagine that the land is your body and the water your chi. In your body, the chi energy flows naturally along the easiest route – a central channel, carrying both rising and descending energy. This energy forms seven areas of intense activity in a line down the centre of your body that can be likened to whirlpools bubbling around rocks in the middle of a fast-flowing river.

In India these energy centres are called 'chakras'. From these seven chakras flow fourteen wide streams of energy known as meridians. Two meridians remain in the torso, six travel to the feet and six to the hands. Each of these meridians has two branches – one branch going to the left hand or foot, and the other to the right.

The flow of chi mirrors the flow of your blood. In the same way that blood flows through smaller and smaller blood vessels until it finally reaches each cell, chi flows through large paths, splitting into smaller and smaller branches until it also reaches each cell. So each cell of your body is nourished by both blood and chi.

THE NATURE OF CHI ENERGY

Chi embodies the invisible, non-physical part of life. It has been described as our soul or spirit, our connection with nature and our consciousness. Just as your blood transports physical nutrients around your body, your chi transports your emotions and ideas to each cell. So, the rush of energy you

CROWN CHAKRA

BROW CHAKRA

THROAT CHAKRA

HEART CHAKRA

SOLAR PLEXUS CHAKRA

SACRAL CHAKRA

BASE CHAKRA

feel when you have an exciting new idea, the physical strength you experience when you are mentally determined, and the way you feel when you are in love – these are all examples of the different physical sensations caused as chi floods into your cells. Highly charged chi makes every cell of your body tingle with life.

IMPROVING THE FLOW

In Japan there are two words to describe the condition of chi energy as it flows around the body: 'kyo' and 'jitsu'. When chi energy is deficient or lacking, it is described as kyo and when there is too much it is known as jitsu. A part of the body that is deficient in energy, or kyo, feels cooler, more hollow and sometimes painful or bruised when pressed. A jitsu area feels swollen, warmer and tense or stiff to the touch.

To help chi flow better through your body you need to disperse chi from the tense jitsu areas and move more energy into the weaker kyo areas. This can be done either by working on the physical structure through which chi flows – the muscles and soft tissue – or directly through the acupressure points.

Each point can be stimulated by pressing deeply while breathing out. If a point feels kyo it will benefit from a long sustained pressure during each slow outbreath as you try to breathe energy deep into it. A more jitsu point will benefit from circular massage and more quick short bursts of pressure as you breathe out, to help disperse the energy.

YIN AND YANG

According to Chinese philosophy, there are two complementary principles at work in the universe: yin and yang. Yin is associated with the feminine and darkness, and yang is associated with the masculine and light. The two principles interact to maintain harmony throughout the universe and to influence everything within it.

Everything, everyone, every state and every quality can be characterized as predominantly yin or predominantly yang. For example, resting is more of a yin state and working is more of a yang state. So, the principles of yin and yang allow you to make basic connections between your environment — the weather, the seasons, the food you eat daily — and your health, and also to describe the essential quality of any phenomena.

A PERFECT BALANCE
The symbol of yin and yang denotes perfect balance and constant movement.

Nothing is static. Everything is always in a state of flux. This ebb and flow can be seen throughout our natural environment: the day (yang) changes to night (yin); summer (yang) changes to winter (yin). Our bodies reflect this natural rhythm: you work (yang) and then you rest (yin); you engage with the world (yang) and then with yourself (yin).

THE SUN AND THE MOON

As the sun comes up, people are naturally physically more active and alert – a more yang characteristic. However, by contrast, during the afternoon most people generally tend to feel more mentally thoughtful and physically passive, and sometimes perhaps even sleepy, and this is more of a yin characteristic.

For some people, the day starts when the moon rises. The moon is essentially yin, creating a more communicative, creative, thoughtful atmosphere than the sun, which is essentially yang and associated with activity and getting things done. The best time for the yin activities of meditation and relaxation is said to be at the time of a new moon. However, sometimes even the moon can influence us to behave in ways that are yang. At the time of a full moon more car accidents and violent crimes occur and there are more disturbances among mentally handicapped patients – these are all more yang effects.

ARE YOU YIN OR YANG?

Everyone is a mixture of both yin and yang characteristics but a person can usually be described as predominantly one or the other. You would describe someone as more yin, for example, if they tended to be relaxed, physically supple, sensitive, creative and imaginative. If someone has become lethargic and depressed, you might describe them as too yin.

You would describe someone as predominantly yang in nature if they tended to be alert, quick, physically active, able to concentrate and pay attention to detail. If someone is tense, irritable, angry or physically stiff and tight, you might describe them as too yang.

In the case of a physical health problem, the cause can be attributed to an extreme of one tendency or the other.

CHECKS AND BALANCES

When someone has a particularly yang experience they often need something yin to counterbalance it. For example, if you eat a lot of dry, salty yang foods at a party you will crave sweet drinks which are comparatively yin. The same is true the other way around: consuming a lot of fruit, salad and sweet drinks, which are more yin, will create a craving for salty, savoury foods.

This balancing effect also applies to the weather. In the autumn and winter the air becomes more cold and damp – both yin qualities. This creates a need for warming foods, such as hot porridge, thick soups and stews, all of which are more yang, to create balance in the body. Conversely, in the spring and summer – as the air becomes warmer and drier, creating a more yang atmosphere – people prefer yin-quality foods that cool the body, such as fruits, salads and drinks.

CREATING YOUR OWN BALANCE

With a simple understanding of yin and yang you can tailor your diet, exercise and lifestyle to make sure that yin and yang remain in balance in your body. For example, if you know you will have to deal with a particularly demanding event next week,

between now and then you should eat more yang foods and do more yang exercises. After the event, you should consume yin foods and undertake yin exercises in order to relax and unwind.

Some of the Do In exercises in this book – for example, pounding, rubbing and shaking – have a more yang, energizing effect; while some – the stretching, kneading and breathing techniques – have a more relaxing, yin quality. Practising these techniques in balance will ensure that you feel both calm and relaxed but also full of energy and vitality.

HEALTHY EATING

One of the great changes in public awareness over the last forty years has been the recognition of the major influence of diet on health. The Health Education Authority, the American Government and the World Health Organization have all published a number of papers confirming the importance of eating a healthy, well-balanced diet based on natural foods.

Medical research has shown that many illnesses – such as heart disease, certain types of cancer, diabetes, arthritis and many other types of what are called degenerative diseases (which is when the body literally degenerates into an unhealthy condition) – can be prevented by eating a healthy diet.

WHAT IS A HEALTHY DIET?

The great debate now is: What is a healthy diet? Most people are agreed that a reduction in saturated fats derived from meat and eggs and all types of dairy foods is a step in the right direction. It is also generally agreed that refined sugars and highly processed foods should be reduced. Instead, more whole grains, fish, beans, fresh fruit and cold-pressed vegetable oils are recommended.

In spite of this, claims and counter-claims appear regularly and the mass of conflicting research and interpretation can paint a confusing picture. In my view, the most sensible approach in such a climate is to look around the world at those societies that have enjoyed long, healthy lives consistently over many generations and discover what their diets have consisted of. Anything less is a risky and unproven experiment.

MODERN MACROBIOTICS

Much of this work has already been done and synthesized into a set of dietary principles called macrobiotics. Originally, macrobiotics was based on a traditional Japanese diet pioneered, after much work, by Doctor Sagan Ishizuka in the 1870s. Since then, the modern macrobiotic diet has been expanded and now represents foods eaten by most of the world's healthiest societies.

Macrobiotics is based on a diet of grains (brown rice, barley, oats, pasta or wholewheat bread), combined with fresh vegetables and beans or fish. This is supplemented by fruits, drinks, nuts, seeds, vegetable oils, seasonings, and a few special foods, such as tofu, miso, shoyu and sea vegetables.

The principles of yin and yang (see page 182) are also taken into account by those following a macrobiotic diet. Some foods have a more warming, strengthening and energizing effect: these are described as yang foods. Others have a more cooling, relaxing and calming effect: these are described as yin foods. A balance between the two types is seen as ideal.

Those following a macrobiotic diet try to tailor it to their particular dietary needs, taking into account their own yin or yang bias, their lifestyle and their daily needs. So, for example, if you intended to embark on some hard physical work outside on a cold day, you would choose to eat a majority of yang foods, such as thick bean soup, fish casserole or oat porridge. Obviously, fruits, salads and juices (all yin foods) would not be as helpful to your body in this particular circumstance.

Conversely, if you wanted to relax outside with friends on a hot, sunny afternoon, you would be well advised to eat more light, yin foods, such as fresh vegetables, juices and salads.

TRY IT OUT

Application of the principles of macrobiotics strengthens your relationship with the planet's natural foods. It ensures that you eat food not only for its taste but also to enhance your physical well-being.

The only way to know whether there is anything to the macrobiotic approach is to do what I did and try it for three months. See how you feel and, if you like it, keep experimenting. After a year or two you will be surprised how aware you have become about food and how well you can make the best choices for your own health.

GLOSSARY

Abdomen Soft area between your lower rib and pubic bone at the front of your body.

Acupressure points Points, known as Tsubos in Japanese, along meridians of chi where you can change the flow of energy most easily.

Bladder Stores fluid bodily waste behind your pubic bone.

Chi A subtle flow of magnetic energy that is present throughout the universe, passing on information from one living entity to another. It carries your thoughts, ideas and emotions within your body.

Do In A Japanese system of self-massage exercises that is based on harmonizing the chi in your meridians and acupressure points.

Gall bladder Stores bile produced by your liver ready to break down fats

during digestion. Situated behind your lower right ribs.

Heart governor Imaginary organ that controls the circulation of chi around your body.

Kidney Two organs behind your lower back ribs that extract fluid waste from your blood.

Large intestine Large-diameter tube that takes solid waste from your small intestine, extracts liquid for re-absorption and sends the remainder to your bowels. It passes up the right side of your abdomen, across just below your ribs and down the left.

Liver Large, multi-task organ that cleans your blood and produces bile for digestion of fats. It is located behind your right lower ribs.

Meditation Emptying and focusing your mind on a single object or word,

enabling you to deeply concentrate on and contemplate something in a relaxed manner.

Meridian A pathway along which chi tends to flow more strongly.

Small intestine A long, thin tube linking your stomach and large intestine in which you absorb your food. It is situated around your navel.

Spleen Cleanses your lymph fluids, which take toxins out of your body.

Stomach Stores food while it is being broken down ready for digestion. This organ is located in between your ribs at the front of your body.

Triple heater Imaginary organ that represents the combining of calories and oxygen to produce heat and physical energy.

ABOUT THE AUTHOR / RESOURCES

SIMON BROWN qualified as a design engineer, having two inventions patented in his name. In 1981 he began studies in Oriental medicine and qualified as a shiatsu therapist and macrobiotic consultant. While studying these healing arts, he studied feng shui with Japanese masters in the USA. Simon Brown was the director of London's Community Health Foundation for seven years, a charity that ran a wide range of courses specializing in the Oriental healing arts. Simon has, since 1993, made feng shui and shiatsu his full-time careers. His clients include well-known celebrities, such as Boy George and large public companies including The Body Shop and British Airways. Simon is a member of the Shiatsu Society.

Consultations with Simon G. Brown

Simon provides a complete feng shui consultation service. Consultations can be arranged to include a site visit or they can all be done by post. These consultations include floor plans with all the feng shui recommendations, a full report including a survey, explanation of the recommendations, your feng shui astrology information for this year and the next three years, your best directions for this year and the best dates to implement the recommendations. Ongoing advice by telephone or e-mail is also included. Simon also provides shiatsu treatments from his London clinic.

Courses with Simon G. Brown

Simon provides a variety of feng shui courses, ranging from one-day introductory courses to a full certificate course with homework and an assessment. He also conducts a range of courses for architects and designers.

Books by Simon G. Brown

Chi Energy Work Book, Carroll & Brown, London, 2003

Choose Your Food to Change Your Mood (written with Steven Saunders), Carroll & Brown, London, 2003

Essential Feng Shui, Cassell & Co, London, 1999

Feng Shui, Thorsons, London, 2001

Feng Shui in a Weekend, Hamlyn, London, 2002

Feng Shui for Wimps, Sterling, New York, 2003

The Practical Art of Face Reading, Carroll & Brown, London, 2000

Practical Astrology by Numbers, Carroll & Brown, London, 2003

Practical Feng Shui, Cassell & Co, London, 1998

Practical Feng Shui for Business, Ward Lock, London, 1998

Practical Feng Shui Solutions, Cassell & Co, London, 2000

Contact Details

Simon G. Brown, PO Box 10453, London NW3 4WD
Tel: +44 (0) 20 7431 9897
Fax: +44 (0) 20 7431 9897
E-mail: simon@chienergy.co.uk
www.chienergy.co.uk

THE ILLUSTRATORS

Dan Fletcher, illustrator of the original edition of this book, has illustrated various books, including Whole Health Shiatsu by my original shiatsu teachers, Shizuko Yamamoto and Patrick McCarty, together with training manuals for companies, including Porsche, Renault and Paris Metro. He can be contacted at: 68a Richmond Road, London sw20 opq; e-mail: dan-fletcher@lineone.net; tel: +44 (0) 20 8946 7745.

Ian Dicks started illustrating twenty-five years ago, after a short spell as an advertising art director. During this time he has worked for most magazines and advertising agencies. He now lives and works in Dorset, in an old undertaker's next to the sea, with his wife, children's illustrator Margaret Chamberlain, and a few happy ghosts.

RESOURCES

UK

The Shiatsu Society
Eastlands Court, St Peter's Road, Rugby, Warks CV21 3QP
Tel: 0845 130450 / Fax: 01788 555052
E-mail: admin@shiatsu.org
www.shiatsu.org

USA

American Organization for Bodywork Therapies of Asia
1010 Haddonfield, Berlin Road, Suite 408, Voorhees, NJ 08043
Tel: (856) 782 1616
E-mail: aobta@prodigy.net

American Shiatsu Association
PO Box 718, Jamaica Plain, MA 02130

Australia

Australian Shiatsu Association
www.australianshiatsuassociation.com.au

Shiatsu Therapy Association of Australia
PO Box 598, Belgrave, Victoria 3160
Tel: (03) 9457 5834
E-mail: staa@mira.net

ACKNOWLEDGEMENTS

Author's Acknowledgements
All my love goes to Dragana, Christopher, Alexander, Nicholas, Michael and Mum for being so special and my greatest source of inspiration to want to write so many books. Thanks to Shizuko, Ohashi, Patrick McCarty, Saul Goodman and Patrick Riley.

Eddison•Sadd Editions

EDITORIAL DIRECTOR Ian Jackson
MANAGING EDITOR Tessa Monina
PROJECT EDITOR Jane Laing
PROOFREADER Nikky Twyman
PRODUCTION Oonagh Phelan and
   Charles James

ART DIRECTOR Elaine Partington
DESIGNER Malcolm Smythe
PHOTOGRAPHERS Stephen Marwood
   and Sue Atkinson
MODELS Emily Outred and
   Alain Li Ko Lun

The image on page 182 is reproduced courtesy of Wellcome Institute Library, London